just jessie

THIS SIGNED EDITION HAS BEEN SPECIALLY
BOUND AND PRODUCED BY THE PUBLISHER.

Dear Target guests,

Target is my go-to place for shopping—or just for a mommy getaway. That's why the next two pages have tips just for Target guests.

Target has the *best* products. I love their Market Pantry food items, and I always have to check out the home department. Target is up with all the trends in home decor, so I have tons of items from the store in my house. I also stock up on their jersey sheets. When it comes to bedsheets, I need to have the best of the best—and Target's jersey sheets are great. And naturally, I could spend hours in the beauty aisle. Some of my favorite brands for beauty come from Target.

Beyond all the products, Target is just a great place to spend time. When I bring the kids, I buy a bag of popcorn for them and a Starbucks latte for me, and we cruise the aisles. My kids never misbehave because there are so many fun things for them to look at. (My children love Target as much as I do; they hang out in the toy department and try to convince me they need all the stuff they've picked out.)

I always end up leaving with more items than I need, but everything is great quality. And I feel good while I'm shopping, which is why Target is my mommy-getaway place, too. Whenever I visit my mom in a little town outside of Atlanta, I leave my kids with her for an hour or two, head straight to the local Target, grab my latte, and let their beautiful, fresh, and fun products take me away.

Whether you need a bar of soap or a break from life, try it yourself sometime! You won't regret it.

Xoxo,
Jessie

MOMMY BREAK

Moms need breaks in order to keep doing all the things they do every day. We're people, too, and we need our own personal time.

I didn't find that going from one child to two was all that hard—because Viv and her brother are seventeen months apart, the whole baby thing was still very fresh when Bubby came into this world. But the shift from two to three children has been a *huge* hurdle. Having an infant who doesn't sleep, a toddler who I'm trying to potty train, and a four-year-old who is becoming her own little person all under the same roof can be really, really exhausting.

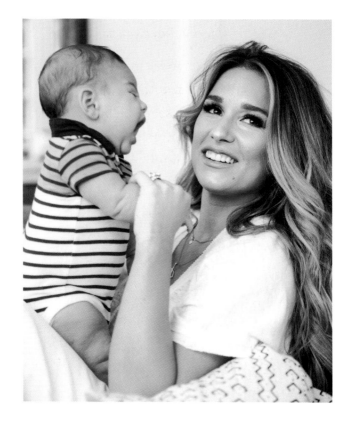

I've always believed in the mommy break, but now that I'm a mother of three, they're a necessity. Here are some of my favorite getaways. I know it's hard, but try to give yourself one of these every week. You'll be a better mom!

* **GET YOUR NAILS DONE:** Go with a sister, a friend, or just by yourself.

* **TAKE A BATH—ALONE:** Tell your husband that you need him to take care of the kids while you head to the bathroom, lock the door,

run a bath, and jack the music up (so you can't hear them call you, which isn't allowed anyway).

* **TAKE A WALK**: Throw on your tennis shoes, put in your earbuds (to listen to music or call a friend or family member), and head out to clear your head. Even walking around the block helps.

* **SCHEDULE A MOMMY'S NIGHT OUT**: Get your other mommy friends on a group text and spearhead a dinner out or cocktails. It's so important to separate the mother from the woman. (This might include helping each other find baby-sitters; there's nothing worse than when one friend can't go because she doesn't have a sitter.)

my top snacks when on the go

* **GRAB THE GOLD**: This is a delicious and filling high-protein oats-and-chocolate bar that's only 190 calories.

* **PREMIER PROTEIN SHAKE**

* **BEEF JERKY**

* **PLANTAIN CHIPS**: Because they are salty and delicious and simple.

* **HOMEMADE HAM-AND-CHEESE ON WHEAT SANDWICHES**: I'll make one, put it in a Ziploc baggie, and bring it with me on my day, just like I'm a kid.

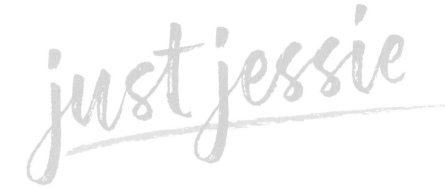

just jessie

MY GUIDE TO LOVE, LIFE, FAMILY, AND FOOD

jessie james decker

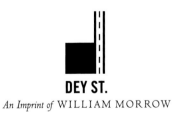

DEY ST.

An Imprint of WILLIAM MORROW

HarperCollins books may be purchased for educational, business, or sales
promotional use. For information, please email the Special Markets Department
at SPsales@harpercollins.com.

FIRST EDITION

Designed by Suet Chong

Library of Congress Cataloging-in-Publication Data has been applied for.

ISBN 978-0-06-285137-6

18 19 20 21 22 LSC 10 9 8 7 6 5 4 3 2 1

I dedicate this book to my fans

who inspired me to write it—

and to my sweet babies.

Y'all are the best thing I've ever done.

I wake up smiling every day

because I get to be your mommy.

contents

introduction

The reason I decided to write this book is because my amazing fans frequently ask me how I do it all. How do I balance my work, family, and personal time? How did I overcome being bullied in school or moving fourteen times before I graduated high school? How am I able to balance being a wife, a new mother, and a friend? What I love about my fans is they aren't afraid to ask. In every meet and greet I do, almost every young girl asks me how I do this or do that. Within those three minutes we have for our picture, I cram in as much advice as possible because it's so important to me. But it's never enough time to say everything I want to.

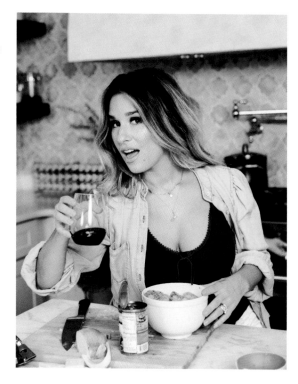

Ever since I was young, dreaming of being a big country star singing to sold-out arenas, I wanted to be that girl other girls could look up to. My main mission has always been to inspire, help, and build confidence in women.

Just Jessie is just that! In telling my story—where I'm from and who I am now—I want women everywhere to know:

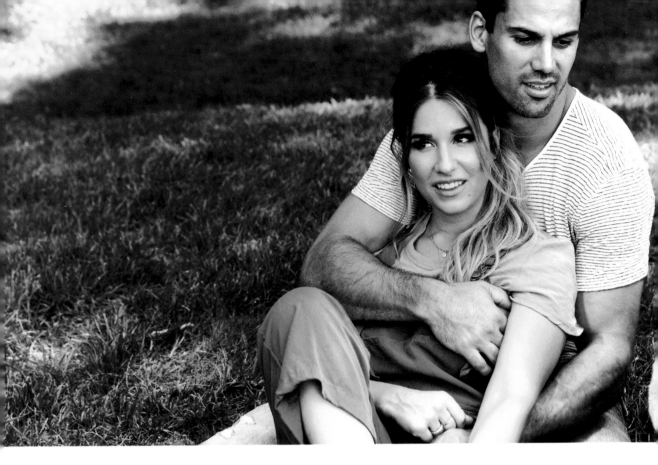

you can do anything you put your mind to, from landing your dream man to losing the baby weight. Whether you're a stay-at-home mom tired from an afternoon of folding laundry or a career woman disappointed by yet another bad date, I've got some easy advice that will lift you up—or at least make you laugh.

I want women to throw off their heels, get into a bubble bath with a glass of wine, and smile or cry with me. I want you to turn the oven to 350 degrees and whip up something delicious with me. I want you to break a sweat with me. And I want you to grab your eyebrow pencil and fill those babies in with me, because we all know how I feel about eyebrows.

We are in this together, and that is why I wrote this book. So grab a warm chocolate chip cookie, lay like broccoli, and enjoy *Just Jessie*.

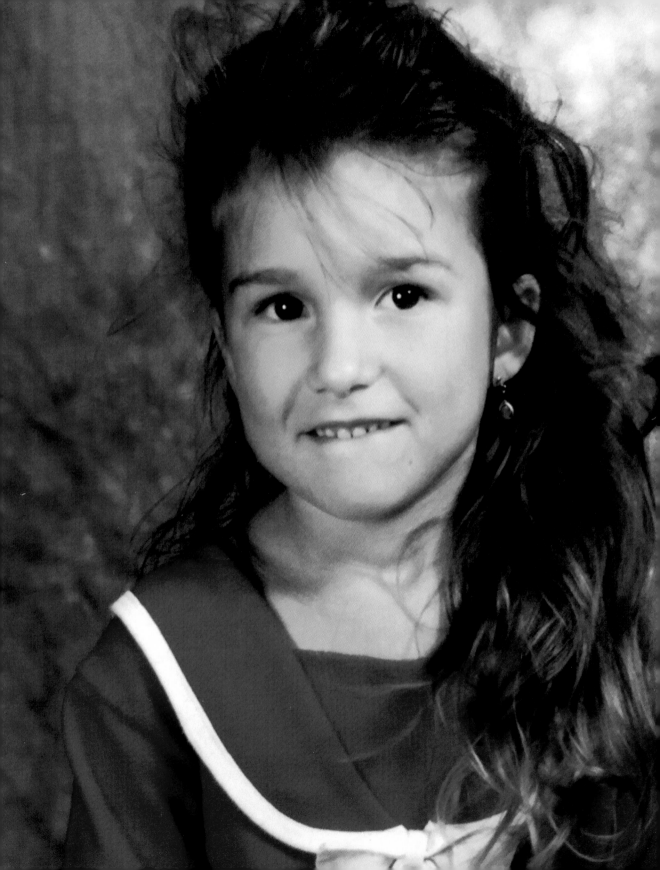

roots and wings

I was born in Vicenza, Italy, at a military field hospital. When my mama set foot on Italian ground at age nineteen, she said it was like coming home. She tells me that when she landed, she felt like dropping to her knees and kissing the ground. Probably because our entire family was from Sicily.

I came into this world faceup. They call that a stargazer, and a stargazer I have remained. Coming out faceup, though, is difficult in the delivery process. I was two weeks late, and my poor mama was on day three of being in labor—and with no epidural. It was so bad they thought we both might not make it. I guess you could say I was a mama's girl before I was even born because I didn't want to come out. A story my mom tells me is that after three days of my refusing to come out, and as a last-ditch effort before an emergency C-section, the doctor propped his foot up on the table and yanked me out. I finally came into the world—all nine and a half pounds of me. My poor mother. My mom even tells me that when she screamed after they cut the umbilical cord, the doctor said, "You aren't supposed to be able to feel that." With her eyes still closed, drenched in sweat, and barely able to speak, she replied, "Well, I did." I guess you could say that's how connected we were and always would be.

Despite the horror of my birth and the fact that she was pretty much on her own when I came home from the hospital, my mom says I was instantly the joy in her life. "Once you were born, I didn't see

anything else but you," she has told me. With my dad busy in the military and the rest of the family miles away, it was just my mom and me. She took me everywhere: to pastry shops, museums, on the bus for hours to see Rome. I received a rosary blessed by the Pope himself. Those are some of her fondest memories.

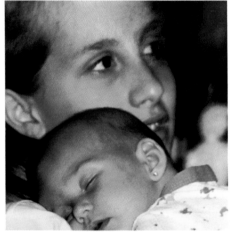

Some of *my* fondest memories are from spending summers with my mama's family in their tiny little country house in a strawberry field in Independence, Louisiana. I can still remember the smell of sweet garlic that always hung in the air, the sound of the air conditioner propped on the window that buzzed throughout the day, and the way walking on the floors would make the whole house shake when you went from one room to the next. I used to perform for all my Sicilian relatives, just as I did for my young mother, who would encourage me in her sweet Louisiana accent by saying, "Sing for Mama."

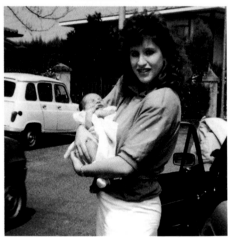

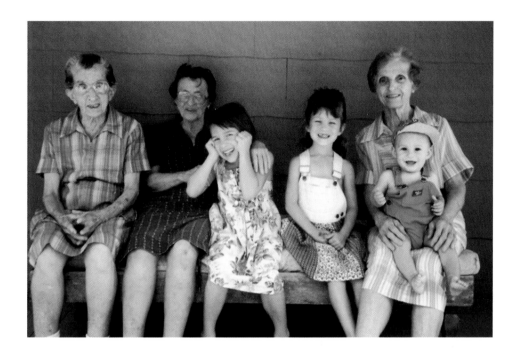

My mama grew up as the youngest of five siblings in Baker, a town an hour away from Independence. Her daddy died when she was four years old, which sent her family into poverty. This was one of the many things that shaped my mother into the person she is today. She was also the most beautiful girl in that town, with golden tan skin and long light brown hair and stars in her big brown eyes. She dreamed of leaving Louisiana and becoming an actress in Hollywood. She wanted more adventure than the little town she grew up in could provide. At eighteen years old, she married my biological father and then a year later moved to Italy, where he was stationed and I was soon born.

FAMILY AFFAIR

From an early age, I was like a little grown-up. "You were not born brand new," my mom would say. Sensitive (maybe overly so) to people's emotions and my surroundings, I never felt like a kid even when I was one. I was more socially aware than other children and had an understanding of adults that was way beyond my age. (My intuition has helped me in my career—whether I'm onstage or in a meeting for my clothing label, I can read the

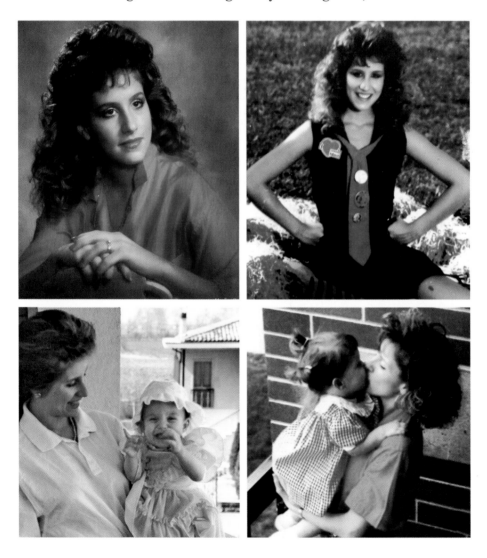

vibe. I might not know how to make a spreadsheet, but I know chemistry and people's energies. That's a skill I was given.)

Even though I was the oldest of my siblings, Sydney, John, and I were a team. As kids, the three of us were very close. Sometimes we would all wind up snuggling in one bed together, something we did even until I was a freshman in high school. Three years apart, Sydney and I enjoyed playing with our Barbies and other games while my brother was still a little baby. And she knew I always had her back. Once when Sydney was in pre-K, she peed in her pants. At that age, parents always keep an extra set of clothes in school. But once her teacher helped her change, she refused to go back into the classroom. Sydney was humiliated at the thought that her classmates would know what happened when they saw her in a different outfit.

"I won't go back in there until I see my sister," she said.

The teacher pulled me out of my class and brought me to Sydney standing in the hallway.

"No one's going to know," I told her gently. "You're all good."

Then I took her little sweet hand and walked her into her classroom. With me by her side, Sydney was fine.

I was a protective big sister, but I never mothered my younger siblings.

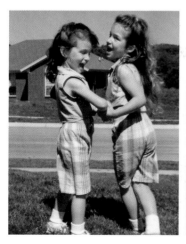 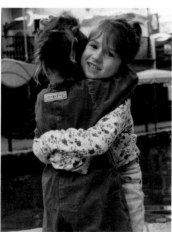 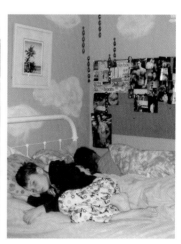

There's a difference. I never felt the need to take care of them in that way. My role was to be a big sister and always be there when they needed me to hold their hand.

I know not everyone has a mom like I do, and I thank my lucky stars for her every day. She's the main reason for a lot of my success, because she always made me feel like I could do anything. And it wasn't just me. She encouraged my sister and brother just as much. Whatever we wanted, she wanted to help us achieve it. For example, John went through a period where he wanted to be a ninja. My mom didn't dismiss his dream as absurd or impossible. Nope, she signed him up for karate and made him a ninja outfit. That's my mom in a nutshell. Whatever our dreams, my mom always figured out a way to make them come true.

I've known I wanted to sing since the moment I formed my first thoughts in my toddler mind. I knew I wanted to perform, entertain, make people smile.

If that's what I wanted, well, Mama was gonna make it happen.

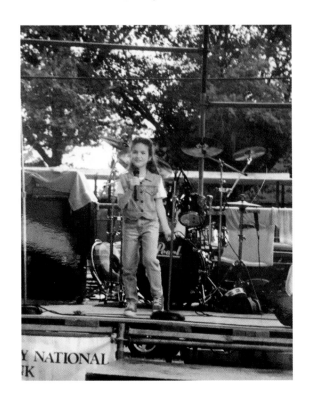

I sang from the time I could walk, but the first time I performed onstage I was nine. It had been my dream for a long time, so my mom found a local talent show in her hometown of Baker, Louisiana.

Dressed in little blue jeans, a blue-jean vest, and red Converse shoes, and with my hair really big and rolled and pushed back in a headband, I got onstage and

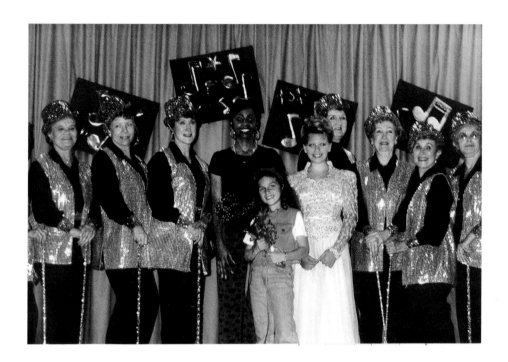

yodeled. That's right, yodeled. My mom had helped me choreograph my dance moves, and I learned to yodel like everything else I sang: by just listening to the music. My mom would buy me tapes, and I would emulate what I heard (which included a lot of LeAnn Rimes).

Well, I won! Not just the children's division but the entire competition, which also had teen and adult divisions. It was the first time in the history of this show that a kid took the grand prize. My success might have been because I was so comfortable onstage (or maybe it was my mom's advice to wink at the judges, which I followed).

Even if I hadn't won, that was it. I had discovered a piece of myself: I was a performer. Like I told my mom right after the show, "I want to do this forever."

BIT BY THE BUG

From then on, I asked my mom to put me in any and every festival or fair where there was a stage and amateurs allowed on it. She drove me all over creation so I could perform.

Whatever the competition, I usually won, which was external validation that I was in the right field. (It would take many years and some hard experiences to learn that internal validation—believing in oneself—is just as important.) As a kid, though, winning signified to me that I was good, that I had a chance at turning this passion into a profession.

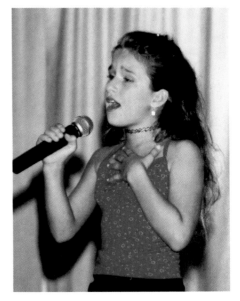

I even won when I entered a competition for amateur rappers and R&B singers, sponsored by the Atlanta R&B/hip-hop radio station Hot 107.9. I was neither a rapper nor an R&B singer, but I entered anything I could because I wanted to sing and get as much practice as possible.

Wearing cheetah-print pants and a full set of braces, I planned to sing the 2001 version of "Lady Marmalade" where Lil' Kim raps in the middle. But as I said, I don't rap. So I found one of the many rappers backstage and asked him if he could come out in the middle of my performance and rap.

"Yeah, I got you," he said.

He didn't.

I went out on the stage and sang my butt off, but when the rap part came, the guy I'd asked to back me up was nowhere to be found. So I rapped myself. I knew the words, and I wasn't about to give up after all that singing and dancing. And you know what? I won the entire contest.

Looking back now, what amazes me—more than the fact that I was a kid who sang mostly country music and won an R&B and rap competition I had no business being in—is how much confidence I had in myself at such an early age. And I know exactly where it came from: my beautiful mama.

My mom was supportive without pushing me. She was the opposite of a stage mother, a phenomenon I witnessed all the time. I felt so sorry for those kids whose moms forced them onstage or obsessed over how they looked. My mom was always clear: "When you don't want to do this anymore, just tell me, and we'll stop. But if you want to keep singing, I'll keep helping you."

She helped me mostly by being my emotional support system, my encourager, my counselor (and my ride everywhere). My mom unknowingly had the instincts to help guide me through this dream. When people suggested I get professional vocal training to help with my craft (because that was the thing to do back then), she didn't think it was a good idea. As a child, I had an impeccable ear and could hear harmonies. She felt like vocal coaches would mess up my natural, God-given talent and make me sound like a pageant singer. She didn't think I needed it; to her, I was perfect just the way I was.

The confidence and security my mom instilled in me are all the more amazing considering that our lives were anything but easy when I was a kid.

BLISSFULLY UNAWARE

My first clue that my family was poor came in elementary school, when my teacher handed out our lunch passes. There were three different-colored cards: one for paid lunch, one for subsidized lunch, and one for free lunch. Mine was *free*. I was confused, because I never lacked for anything—at least not that I knew of.

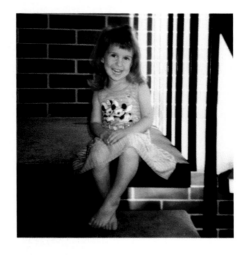

My suspicions about our economic status were confirmed in fifth grade, when I started at a private school. We had moved to San Antonio, Texas, where our local public school was failing. Mom, a clever woman who never settled for anything but the best for her children, applied for financial aid and got us into a Catholic school.

The first day of school, an administrator took me into the cafeteria, where there was an enormous locked armoire. She opened up what turned out to be a lost and found filled with uniforms. The lady pulled out clothes in my size, including a pair of shorts covered in acid stains (that I later hid by tying a sweatshirt around my waist). Going to a fancy private school confirmed it: we didn't have any money. We couldn't afford new uniforms or lunch boxes filled with fancy packaged Capri Suns and other little store-bought snacks that all the other kids had.

I'm not complaining. On the contrary, I never felt disappointed or less-than in any way growing up. My mom told me later on as a young adult about when times were especially tight. My parents both went to college at Boise State after we returned from Italy and had a summer back in Louisiana to try to figure out their next step. I can't imagine what it was like for my mom with little children, a full course load, and a job to try to keep food on the table. During that period, our family had to go on food stamps. Despite the government assistance, there were times my mom didn't eat for days, because there simply wasn't enough money for food and diapers. I didn't know it at the time, though, because I always had a full belly.

She didn't have much help as she struggled to survive. (Ultimately, my parents divorced when I was eleven—around the time we were living in San Antonio, where my mom, who earned her degree in communications, landed a job in television.) Again, I didn't know that at the time, because I never saw my mom sad. She never expressed that there was anything wrong. It was the opposite. Picking us up from school, putting dinner on the table, or tucking us into bed, she was always very happy and bubbly.

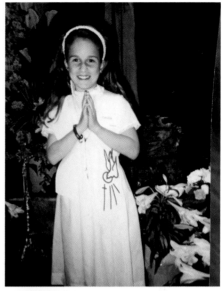

My mother did everything she could possibly do to nurture her children. Food on the table was just the start. She figured out how to get us into the best schools and support us in going after what we wanted in life. Most of all, we always had love. She gave us so much love that we never felt deprived. Nothing was handed to me as a kid, but nothing was missing either.

Now that I'm a grown-up with a family of my own, if I'm ever going through a hard time, I always remember how my mom kept such a positive attitude in much more trying

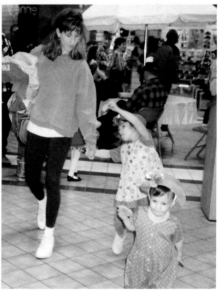

circumstances. If she could keep a smile on her face and be so joyful, there's no excuse for me to be grumpy when I have been so blessed. From my creativity to my work ethic to my family values, everything I know I learned from my mom.

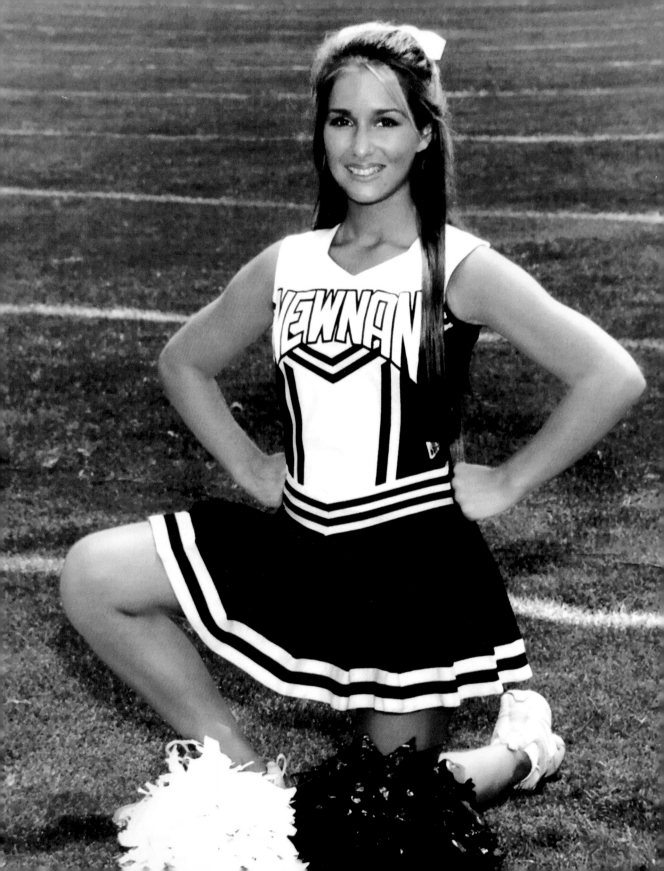

always the new kid

*I*recently counted all the places I lived growing up and came up with fourteen different towns by the time I graduated from high school. We moved around a lot. One year, we moved two times (which meant two different schools).

We moved the most when I was little, because my biological father kept getting stationed at different military bases or landing jobs in different areas. My mom's career in television took us around the country as well.

More than moving to a new town, the biggest change came in fifth grade, when my parents divorced—and shortly after, my mama got remarried to my stepdad, Steve.

That wasn't just the beginning of a new life for my mom. Steve is my family too. For the last seventeen years, this kind and generous man has been a father to me and then a grandfather to my children. All of our lives became more wonderful when he entered them. But my mom's marriage to Steve didn't end our moving around as they relocated for work and to be together.

I was always the new kid and that was never easy. There was nothing worse than arriving at a new school. With each step closer, the pit in my stomach would grow bigger as if something horrible waited for me inside. As I entered my classroom, a cold chill and goose bumps would sweep over me. With the other students staring at me and whispering, I would study the room, hoping to make contact with a pair of kind eyes, to find someone to welcome me or at least have lunch with. Most of the time, I wound up eating lunch alone.

The same scenario happened over and over again. Being new, pretty, and overly nice in my desperation for acceptance was not a good combination. As a kid, I was a constant target.

I never felt accepted in school. *Never.* To this day, I still have weekly nightmares about the first day at a new school: the faces, the whispers, the chill on my skin. School just wasn't a safe place for me. Georgia, Louisiana, Texas—it didn't matter. My school days were spent watching the clock and waiting for the bell to ring so I could get the heck out of there.

Even the teachers were not the best to me growing up. I had some great choir teachers, but there were also some pretty bad ones, including one who rejected me when I auditioned for *Annie* in elementary school. I don't mean I didn't get the lead role; I didn't get *any* role. Here I was winning singing competitions up and down the state, and my own school choir teacher didn't think I had what it took to be an orphan or Sandy the dog or even a tree.

There was a similar incident at one school where you had to audition to perform at the talent show. I belted out Janis Joplin's version of "Me and Bobby McGee." This was a song I frequently performed in my sets, so I nailed it. I had every person in the room staring in amazement because of my raw talent at such a young age. Afterward, we were all told to wait in the hallway while they decided who would be allowed to perform. When the teacher posted the sheet of paper with all the names listed, mine wasn't on it. The girl who clogged before me made it—but not me doing my best mini-Janis.

In fifth grade, when I was attending the private school in San Antonio, the difference in economic status between my peers and me became apparent. "Why do your clothes have holes in them?" girls would ask me. "How come you don't swim at the country club?"

Whether it meant wearing the big bows they all had in their hair or the fancy socks with the frills, I so badly wanted to fit in. But I didn't have any of those things. I had the clothes on my back and a warm house to live in, which I thought was good enough, but clearly they weren't, according to these girls. Sometimes I found myself lying to try to make people like me. I said stupid things, like I had a housekeeper, all in an

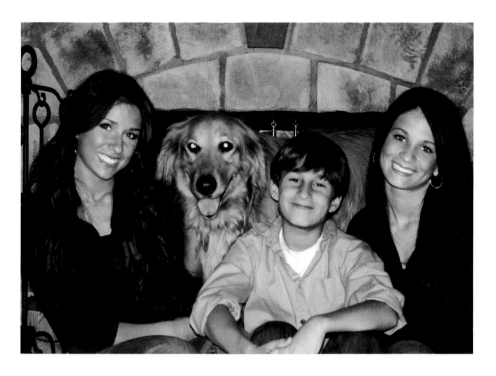

effort to be more in line with the rich popular girls. I'm not a great liar. Nobody bought it.

However, all of that was child's play compared to what happened to me when we arrived in Newnan, Georgia, just as I was entering junior high.

We had been living in Peachtree City, Georgia, for about a year, because Steve had taken a job with Delta Air Lines. After the terrorist attacks of September 11, 2001, Steve decided to return to the military full-time. My mom also got a job in Atlanta, hosting a real estate show called *Atlanta's Best New Homes*. So they settled on Newnan, which allowed them both to commute to their jobs.

Newnan was a beautiful town with a very beautiful school (country star Alan Jackson was a graduate). Large and cream colored, perched on a hill

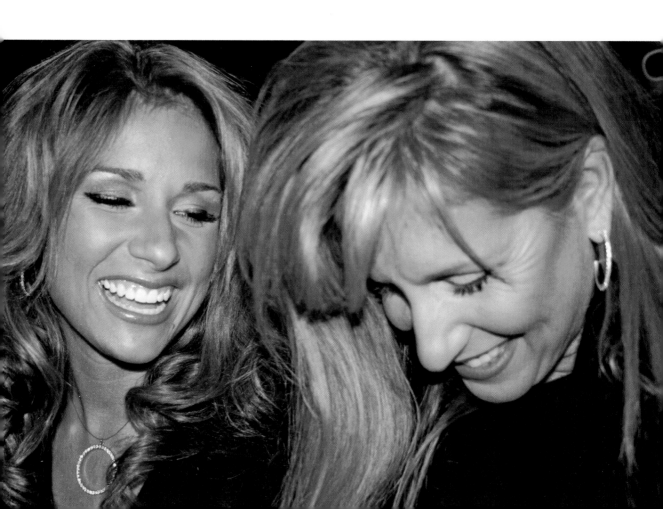

covered in green grass and trees, the school exuded a classic air. It was the kind of school you look at as you drive past with your husband and smile at each other, knowing you both hope your kids will attend one day. It looked like a school out of a movie. And for me, the movie was a horror flick. The halls, when I think about them, still haunt me to this day.

Newnan was filled with the meanest girls. They were on a whole other level. In this cliquey, wealthy town, parents had grown up together, and grandparents too. Meanwhile, *we* blow into town. When my smoking-hot mom picked me up at school, I saw how the other moms looked her up and down with a combination of jealousy and disdain. Unbothered, my mom breezily asked me, "Hey, how was your day at school?" She wasn't worried about the stares. I wish I could have been so cool, but it wouldn't be long before my classmates made me feel like the un-coolest person in the world.

SUCKER

My first traumatic experience in Newnan happened when I had been at the school for only a couple of months. It started when a boy invited me to his birthday party. I didn't really know anyone, but it felt special to be included. Apparently he was a part of the cool crowd, which ruled not only the school but also the town. I got ready for the party by throwing on a pair of old blue jeans and a long-sleeved black cotton top with a big star in front. Technically the shirt was a pajama top, but I thought I could get away with it.

When I arrived at the very imposing house with a circular driveway and huge pool, I was nervous. But the boy who invited me made me feel welcome by being so friendly at the party. I started to relax until about a half hour later, when a group of girls huddled together started laughing and pointing at me. Then one of them approached me and asked, "Where'd you get your top from?" I froze as she pulled the back of my shirt so she could look at the tag. For a moment I thought they might be trying to be nice. But as soon as she walked away, I felt something heavy in my hair. When I reached back with my hand to touch the back of my head, I felt something sticky and wet. It was a lollipop she had sucked and then stuck into my hair, which was now all tangled.

My face turned bright red. I was sick to my stomach. *How* could someone do this? *Why* would someone do this? When I looked back at the girls, they were all laughing at me.

The only doubts I ever had about myself growing up stemmed from my peers. I never understood how girls could be so mean. I literally did not understand—because I grew up with the sweetest mother in the world. My mom made us feel so special that I took it for granted everyone would love me—or at least not hate me.

When my mom picked me up from the party, I was crying and told her everything that had happened. Hugging me close, she explained that "obviously their mommies and daddies didn't treat or teach them well or they wouldn't be so mean." She always tried to help me understand the world through her positive outlook. But Mom also let me know I shouldn't worry. "One day you're going to leave them all in your dust," she said with a smile.

Maybe so, but I still had a long road ahead of me before that would happen.

SLOPPED

With the start of high school, my troubles only got worse. By fourteen, I had developed D-cup boobs, which made me look more like twenty.

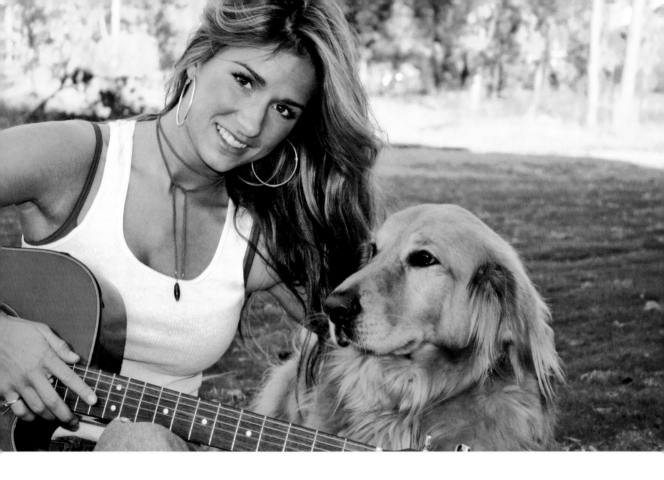

While everyone else in school played it safe in Abercrombie & Fitch 24/7 (which we couldn't afford unless it was on sale), I would experiment with styles. Sometimes I would even cut up old clothes to make new fashions out of them. I had highlighted hair down to my hips and always sported a tan. I didn't look like your typical fourteen-year-old at that school—a fact that was made clear to me.

When I was still a brand-new freshman at Newnan High, I met a girl named Laney who befriended me. A little more than a month after the start of school, Laney invited me to her house for a birthday sleepover party. I was nervous, considering my past experiences with kids at school, but I reassured myself it'd be okay. Laney was one of my only real friends at the time.

The night started out fun—we watched scary movies and ate a lot of snacks. Then Annie, one of the girls at the party, realized she had forgotten her overnight bag and called her older sister Heather to bring it to her. About a half hour later, headlights shone through the windows. "Let's go outside to get the bag!" one of the girls suggested. We were all standing around and 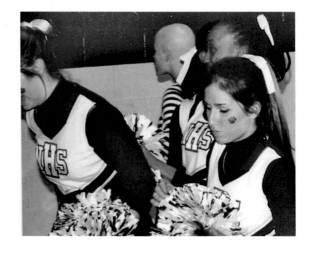 chatting while Annie grabbed her bag, when suddenly someone jumped out of the bushes and dumped a bucket of something cold and wet over my head.

It was just like the scene in *Carrie* where Sissy Spacek is covered in pig's blood after winning prom queen. Except it wasn't blood; it was a bucket of old food and other gross stuff the assailant had been saving for just the right moment to dump on me. I stood there soaked and in shock. I didn't know the girl who had jumped out of the bushes; I had never seen her before, although clearly she went to our school, because Laney shouted at her by name to leave. Laney and the rest of the girls walked me into the house. I was shaken but didn't cry. Even though the girls at the party that night showed compassion for my pain, I was numb from the kind of abuse that had already been heaped upon me. In the shower trying to wash all the slop off me, I thought, "Why does this keep happening?" I had never even seen this girl before. Had she been plotting this? What had I done to inspire her attack? As I dried off, something inside me shifted. I decided then and there I was done trying to fit in.

I had dreams that were so much bigger than the drama of school. I wasn't interested in drinking (even though I went to one party freshman year and held a beer can to appear cool). I was done with the stupid girl gossip and any other ridiculous stuff. If that made me seem stuck-up to the other kids, well, that's a price I was willing to pay.

From then on, I had my eye on the one and only prize that mattered: becoming an entertainer. With this mind-set, I utilized every single tool school provided to educate myself on what was really important to me. So I took graphic design in order to learn how to create T-shirts and logos for one day when I would have my own merchandise at my concerts or maybe even a fashion line. After my extracurricular class on broadcasting development, which I took to learn how to stand in front of a camera and read a teleprompter, I pitched my teacher an idea to start an entertainment news show as part of the school's morning lineup. Every morning at my high school, the TVs in the classrooms played the weather and a list of the activities and deadlines scheduled for the day. My teacher went for it, so every day I wrote and aired pieces on the latest pop culture news, from Nick Lachey and Jessica Simpson's divorce to the trend of low-rise jeans. I was a one-woman version of E!

HOMECOMING

In an odd twist of fate, I won homecoming court my sophomore year. The popular kids, who had it out for me, were in reality a minority in the two-thousand-student school (even if they ruled it with an iron fist). I think the choir vote put me over the top. Either way, the cool crowd wanted me to regret that I had been chosen.

When it comes to homecoming, at Newnan High they do it up. If

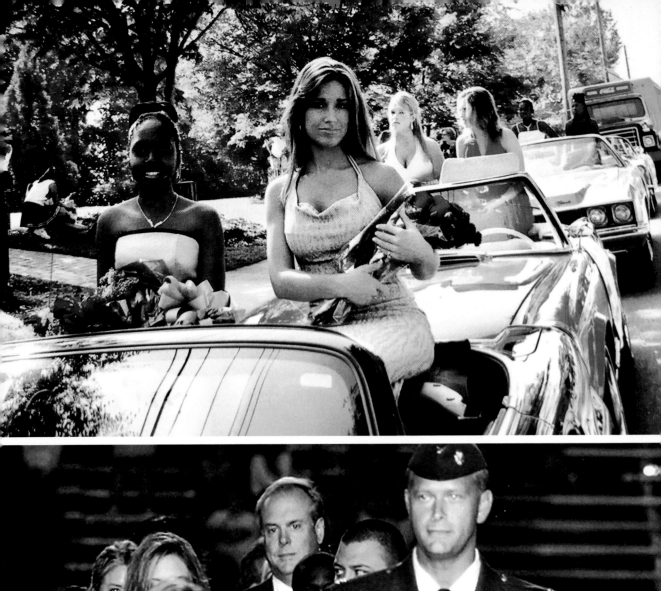
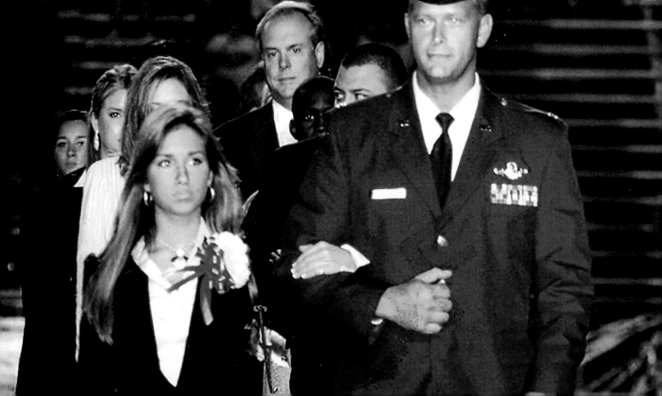

you've ever watched *Friday Night Lights* you get the idea: football and lots of drama. It starts with a parade where the homecoming court rides in sitting in convertibles. Right before the parade, a kid at school broke ranks by telling me that the senior girls had come up with a plan to egg me as I drove by.

I didn't know what to do. I wanted to renounce the title and hide under a rock, but that wasn't possible. Mostly I was sad to be the object of such ridicule. My mom and dad went right to the principal, who decided to have golf carts ride on either side of my car to thwart the plan. I felt sick to my stomach as I drove by the seniors, eggs in hand, and watched their faces drop.

I took heart, however, in the thought that at least the worst of it was over. Halftime began, and the freshman court walked out one by one, each girl on the arm of her dad. Next up was the sophomore court. My turn.

Steve, in his air force dress blues, looked so handsome and proud as he waited for my name to be called.

"Jessica James," the announcer said.

We started to walk, and just then the hairs on the back of my neck stood up (my body feels danger before my eyes see it). The entire student body in the surrounding bleachers started to boo me—the loudest roar of boos I have ever heard to this day. I kept walking forward, pretending I didn't notice but sick to my stomach, because what else could I do? My sweet dad rubbed my back in support.

I wish I could say that I had a confident, screw-you attitude, but in that moment I so badly wanted to be accepted I felt physically ill. I wanted to cry. I wanted to tell myself that what I heard was wrong. But it was clear. One of the senior girls had gotten the entire student body to boo me.

As soon as we left the field, I just wanted to go home. I didn't want to finish watching the game. I didn't even want to talk about what happened. The ride home with my family was quiet. The next day my mom had a little chat with me, and as always she knew the right thing to say.

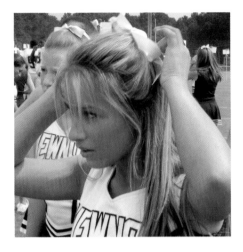

"You don't need these people. In a few years, they'll mean nothing to you. I promise you'll never think about them again." Then she repeated her go-to line to me: "Leave 'em in your dust."

I wanted to heed my mother's words more than anything, and yet I was equally desperate to know why the other girls hated me so much they were willing to publicly humiliate me. I had to believe that God had a plan—that he didn't want me to get wrapped

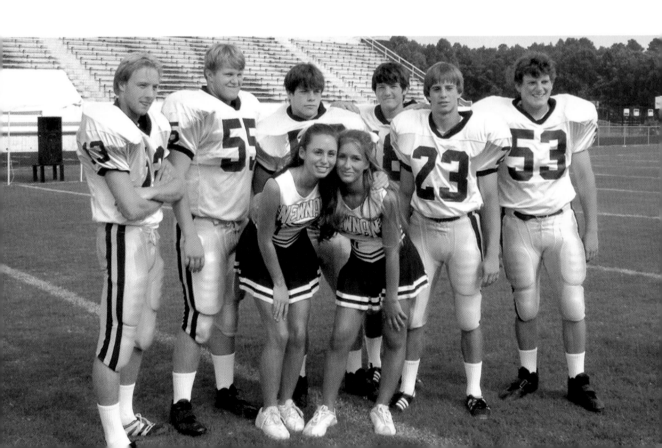

up in the high school social scene, which would have just distracted me from my larger goals.

Unfortunately, the torture didn't stop there. I got in fights in the parking lot and was told to watch my back between classes because someone with scissors was ready to cut my hair, which fell down to my hips. In health class, I thought the girl behind me, who let me borrow a sheet of paper on the first day of school, was my friend—only to find out she'd created a website called the I Hate Jessica James Club, where you could write your reason for hating me. It got so bad that I started keeping my head down between classes and sometimes pulling up my hoodie so no one could get me. Even my high school boyfriend, Thomas, who was my first love, ended up breaking up with me because he wasn't able to handle defending me to his popular friends. I was *the* target at that school. Anyone who attended Newnan High at the same time I did will tell you that it was even worse than I'm describing it.

We wound up living in Newnan for five long years, the longest I had ever lived anywhere in my life. My dad had been commuting to work in Warner Robins, two hours each way, for years. But after my mother quit her TV show job, it didn't make sense to be in Newnan anymore. I couldn't have been happier. "Thank you, Jesus," I thought. "We're getting out of this town!"

When we arrived in Warner Robins, a military town, I was entering my senior year. So although the kids, who came from all over the country and had moved around a lot like me, were much more accepting, I still kept my head down and focused on my dreams of becoming a country singer.

It wasn't like I didn't talk to the other students; I'm always kind to the people around me. I just didn't go out of my way to try to make friends. I didn't hang out with anybody outside of school (I didn't go to

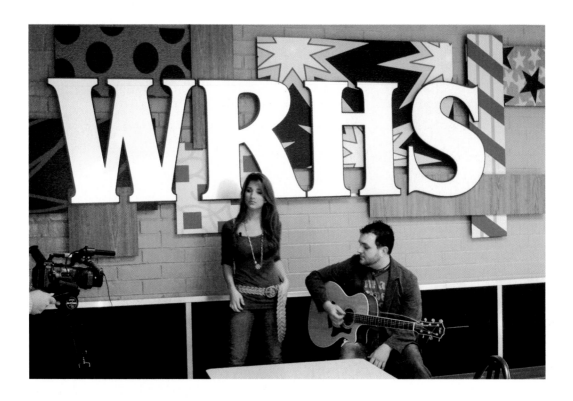

one single party my senior year), and I ate lunch by myself every day. But this time by choice. I wasn't necessarily trying to disappear, but I wasn't trying to show up to anything either. I think I had been hurt so much that I just didn't want to put myself out there.

I viewed school as a job. Get in, get it done, and get out. I had only two credits left to complete, so I didn't have a hard task ahead of me. My senior year was pretty much all fluff, but I made the best of it. I took two graphic arts classes, because by this time I knew I wanted to be a designer someday. I also took two PE classes—an aerobics class and just a regular old gym class—because it's never a waste of time to get your fitness on.

By my senior year, I was doing so much in terms of my music career I had plenty to occupy me outside of school. I entered the My Grammy Moment contest, where unknown performers from across the nation send in tapes to the Recording Academy (formerly the National Academy of Recording Arts and Sciences) for the chance to sing with a big musical artist at the Grammys. That year it was Justin Timberlake. While I didn't wind up doing a duet with J. T., I did make the top five in the whole country and was flown out to LA and put up in a hotel and everything. I made the local newspaper like some kind of little celebrity. I was also

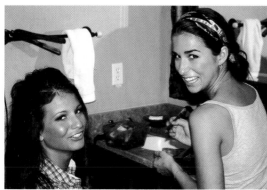

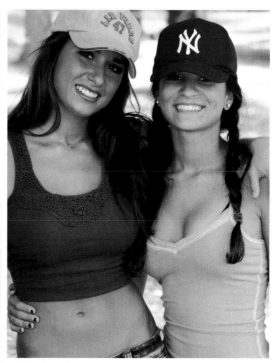

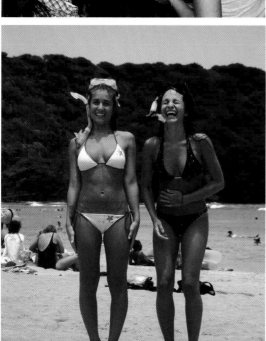

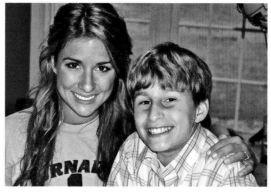

going back and forth to Nashville all the time on weekends with my mom, trying to meet and work with professionals in the music industry. So, yeah, school was an afterthought.

That's why it came out of nowhere when I was nominated for homecoming queen my senior year. It was even more surprising than when I was at Newnan, because back then at least I made an effort (an unsuccessful effort, but I'd tried).

Whatever the reason for my nomination, I was expected to campaign for votes by making posters, passing out candy, and telling kids in the hallways, "Make sure you vote for me for queen!" Well, I definitely wasn't doing any of that.

My little sister, Sydney, wasn't having it. "If you're not going to," she said, "I am."

Sydney, who was in ninth grade, hustled. She made so many posters and flyers, handed out so much candy, and repeated over and over, "Vote for my sister! Vote for my sister!"

During homecoming court, both my parents walked me. They were so proud of me no matter what happened. Right before they called my name, though, my dad whispered, "You're going to win, you know?"

"No, I'm not!" I whispered back.

Then they said my name; I had been named homecoming queen of my senior year.

There were so many ninth graders at the school they had their own separate building. I'm pretty sure

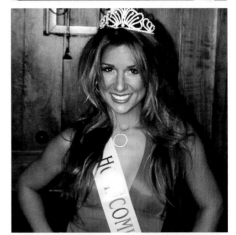

WHERE DO YOU SEE YOURSELF 10 YEARS FROM NOW?

"10 years from now, I will be a well known county artist living in LA or Nashville with my Rockstar husband headlining my own tour and selling lots of records. I will also be involved in many charities and fundraisers to give back to my town and state."
–Jessie James

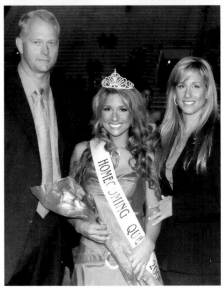

the ninth-grade vote secured my title. The ninth-grade PE coach confirmed it when he said, "You better thank your sister, 'cause she's the reason you won."

My mom said, "This is God's way of giving you one really great moment for high school."

Maybe so, but Sydney also had a huge hand. It was the sweetest thing. She's such a good sister.

In my senior yearbook, to the question of where I saw myself in ten years, I wrote, "I'm going to be a well-known country singer, living in LA or Nashville with my rock star husband."

Two weeks after graduating high school, we packed up a U-Haul with all my stuff and my dad drove me and my dog, Lulu, to Nashville to make it happen.

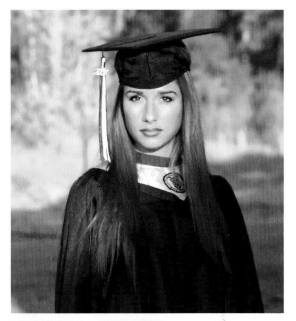

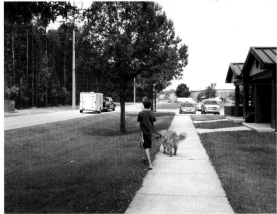

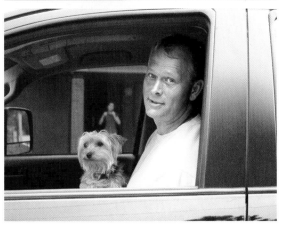

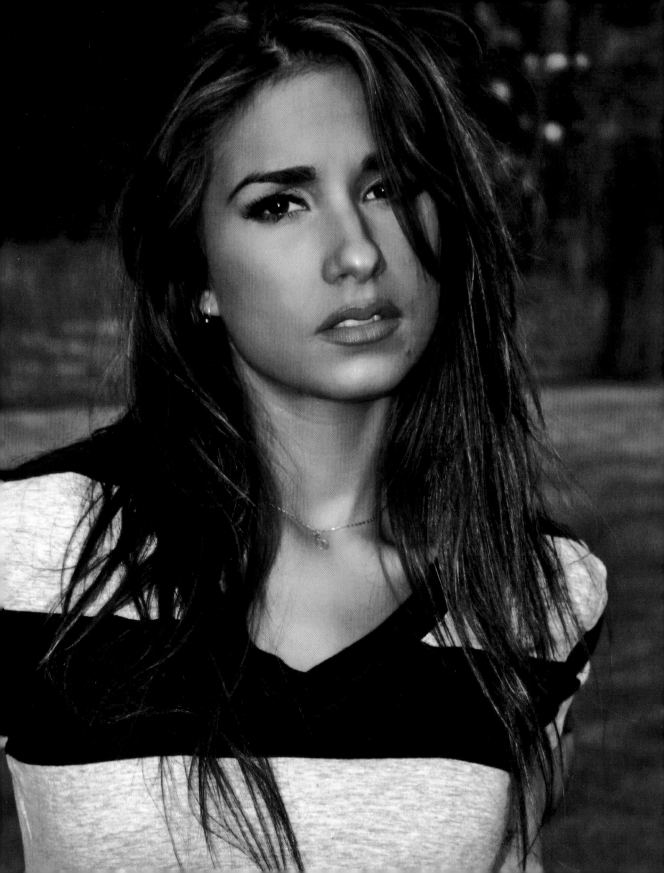

signed, sealed, and lost

Nashville wasn't entirely new to me when I moved there after high school. Ever since I was fifteen—after a songwriter heard me doing my Janis Joplin routine around the pool while on vacation in Florida and said, "You really need to come to Nashville"—I'd made the five-hour drive from home to the heart of country music regularly. Or rather, my mom did that drive about a million times while I sat in the passenger seat singing along to the radio.

My voice got me a lot of meetings with writers and producers, but the person who would play a big role in helping me get my start in the business was someone I met right at home in Georgia!

It started when one of my choir friends (boy, they were responsible for a lot of good stuff in my life) invited me to his grandfather's golf course, where the country music singer Billy Currington was going to perform after a tournament. I stood in line at the meet and greet, but as soon as it was my turn to take a picture with the boyish country star, I said, "One day, we're going to be on the same label, and I'm going on tour with you."

I was all of seventeen.

"Oh really," he said with his coy smile.

When I sang for him, though, he changed his tune. His eyes lit up, and the wheels started turning. "I'm going to set you up with a publisher who can help you," he said, "because I think you got it, girl."

Billy himself was just getting his rhythm going on country radio with his first number one. (He now has eleven number ones on the *Billboard* Hot Country or Country Airplay chart and multiple platinum records.) I'm forever indebted to him for introducing me to Carla Wallace, who is still my publisher to this day, because that changed everything for me. He really believed in me, and we have a special friendship I will always cherish and be grateful for.

Carla, a sassy country lady who has an incredible ear for talent, runs a publishing company called Big Yellow Dog Music, and since the moment I met her when I was seventeen, she has been one of my biggest and most consistent supporters. Music-wise, I don't know where I would be without her. She's not just a publisher for songwriters; she's an artist developer, responsible for the likes of Meghan Trainor, Maren Morris, and so many others. She goes above and beyond her role as a publisher, pouring her whole heart and soul into the people she believes in.

When I moved to Nashville to pursue music full-time, Carla set me up with lots of writing appointments. That's where you and another writer meet at a songwriter house. Those are mini-businesses all over Nashville with cozy writers' rooms where you work on songs for Blake Shelton or Carrie Underwood or anyone who's looking for a song.

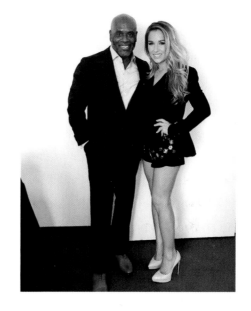

I wrote *all* the time. Ultimately, I wrote enough songs that one of my demos ended up in the hands of a talent scout for Mercury Records/Island Def Jam, and I went to New York City to audition for the famous music executive Antonio "L.A." Reid.

I had studied the faces of all the country music label execs online so that if I ever ran into anyone, I would know whom I was dealing with. But I never educated myself on the pop side of the world, and boy is that a good thing. L.A. Reid is one of the most powerful label legends of our generation, but I did not know who he was at the time and had no nerves leading up to the meeting.

I still remember my first time flying up to New York City and being put up at a fancy hotel, my eyes filled with stars and excitement. As I walked into L.A.'s office, I could tell the A&R guy, David Gray, and the president of Mercury, David Massey, were very nervous. Their anxiety was written across their faces. Singing for the boss man was my last hurdle to signing with the big label. I entered with my hair big and rolled beauty queen style, my white denim shorts, and my navy tube top, and there was L.A. himself sitting behind his desk in this massive corner office with windows that exposed the entire city of Manhattan. I can still remember the smell of his fancy candles, and to this day if I ever pass one in Barneys, I send him a pic to let him know I'm thinking of him.

The song I auditioned with was called "My Cowboy," which I had recently written with Jamey Johnson and Randy Houser. John Rich produced it. These three men were like big brothers to me in Nashville and helped me tremendously. I had a CD with no vocals to use as background music, which L.A.'s assistant Ira put in the player. No sooner did the whip and banjo begin to play than I started to sing the first verse. L.A. stared at me with a frown. He looked over at Ira and told him to stop the CD. He then glared at me and said, "Are you lip-synching?"

Shocked at his question, I answered, "No, sir."

He told his assistant to press play again and asked me to be quiet so he could check. . . . No vocals. L.A.'s face lit up, and he told me to sing again. I did. He was so excited, he got up from behind his desk and started dancing. I kept singing and moving my body from side to side. After the song was over, he asked me, "You hungry?" Before I could answer, however, he said, "Let's go to dinner."

Another powerful label president caught wind that I was about to be signed to Island Def Jam, and he decided to hop on a plane to try to convince me to sign with him. L.A. flew my parents in from Georgia and put me up in the Hamptons to hide me away (with no phone service) until the deal was done. And like that, at nineteen, I was officially signed. I was on my way. When my first album, *Jessie James,* debuted in the summer of 2009 at number twenty-three on the *Billboard* 200, it was a dream come true. Its lead single, "Wanted," went gold!

Big Yellow Dog wasn't just responsible for my landing a record deal. The publishing company is also where I met my first friend in Nashville. I was at the office one day to meet Carla when a friendly brunette with warm brown eyes and a big smile introduced herself. She was Hallie Harris, a song plugger at Yellow Dog. "Let's go to dinner," she said. And pretty much instantly she became a girlfriend of mine.

Hallie came into my life exactly when I needed her and took me under her wing. She is totally nonjudgmental, which is ironic since, growing up, Hallie was the consummate cool girl. She was a debutante with so much confidence and so many friends. Several years older than me, she took me in—literally and figuratively. Not long after we met, I moved in with Hallie, who showed me how to be a grown-up in little ways, like how to tip on a food bill. She also let me live with her rent-free for almost two years.

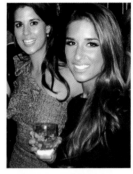

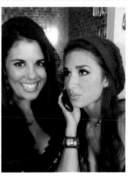

Hallie's generosity, which gave me a sense of security, went beyond a free place to stay. I was still very wounded from school. My experience with high school bullies was so traumatic that it carried over into my adulthood. For the first few years after graduation, I was unable to be around group social situations without having an anxiety attack. I was sure that people were pointing at me, and I would begin to shake and struggle to hold back my tears.

Meanwhile, Hallie was a very popular and social person. Whenever she hosted a party or had a few friends over, I would either go to my room and shut the door or go to a movie by myself. I was so scared that everyone hated me. I couldn't relax around strangers and just hang out, have a glass of wine, and talk. The idea alone made me feel uncomfortable. I couldn't understand my own emotions, so I did the only thing I could: shut down.

To her credit, Hallie never pushed me or treated me like I was strange. Instead she invited me to join her friends, and when I invariably said no, she gently replied, "Okay." But it was clear I was suffering from post-traumatic stress disorder from my many years of bullying and I was not ready to be around my peers. It made for a lonely life. For the very first time, I was out on my own, living in a new city and trying to make a go of a tough career. On top of that, Steve was transferred to Hickam Air Force Base in Hawaii, so my entire family now lived more than four thousand miles away.

Isolated and insecure, I was the perfect target for the wrong boyfriend. Enter Angelo.

Okay, you can probably guess Angelo is not his real name. He was one of the many music producers I was introduced to when I first arrived in Nashville. He wasn't particularly good-looking, but he had a swagger about him that came from the fact that he was so musically gifted. I was attracted to his talent. Because I loved music so much, I thought I needed to date it—and I pretty much talked him into being my boyfriend. Never a good start.

From the get-go it was a bad relationship. He was a master at making me feel bad or that I owed him everything. Once while in the car, coming back from dinner, I asked him one of those silly things you do when you're looking for a little compliment: "Do you think I'm the prettiest girl in the world?"

He paused and then said, "Well, let me think about it."

What the heck was there to think about?

Finally, after way too long, he said, "My ex Jenny was really pretty. But I guess I'd have to say you." (If I were to ask my husband, Eric, that question right now, he wouldn't even flinch.)

His commentary on my appearance didn't just affect me personally but also professionally. One of his common refrains was that I shouldn't wear makeup. Now, I know a lot of women are reading this and thinking, "What's so bad about that?" It was actually a manipulative tactic on his part, just like his talking me out of working with other music professionals. It got to the point where I was trying not to look like a star. That might be great for some women, but I was trying to be a country music star. I needed to be glamming it up, not wearing sweats and a topknot.

I learned that lesson the hard way when at a meeting one of the execs at my label said, "Jessie, what are you doing? When you show up to this office, I need you to look like a star. You look like you just rolled out of bed."

Looking back, I can see now that Angelo was trying to keep me down, because if I thought I was Miss Thing, then I would realize I didn't need him. At the time, though, I was so mixed up and lost I would have done practically anything he told me to.

I lacked confidence in all areas of my life. My emotions were controlled by an unloving man. Meanwhile, my musical career was controlled by my label—and as time went on, I didn't like the direction they were taking it in. For my debut album, they positioned me as a pop music vixen, a guy's girl, someone who did *not* appeal to women. I knew better. Sometimes you should listen to the people around you, but there are a lot of times you have to listen to your inner voice. And I didn't listen.

When music videos from my first record played on CMT and its website, the comments from women were so nasty and so *many* that the site's administrator had to disable the comments section. I was accused of being a slut and worse. It was just horrible.

I was immediately catapulted back to high school. Just like the girls in school, I felt like the women upset over my videos wouldn't judge me so harshly if they could get to know me—the real me. But nobody wanted to give me a chance. No girls wanted to be fans of mine, because they couldn't see past me parading around in Daisy Dukes.

My career was "taking off." So much so that I landed the spot opening for the Jonas Brothers, who were huge at the time. And yet I found myself underneath the stage in a New Jersey arena, crying by myself right before I was about to perform. I was supposed to be having the time of my life, but the reality couldn't have been further from that. (I ultimately got kicked off the Jonas Brothers tour, because the concertgoers were mostly girls and, well, girls hated me.)

My mental state began to manifest physically. I lost a lot of weight, getting down to 102 pounds. While I had been a honey blond my whole life, I began to dye my hair dark, dark brown. I think it was a futile attempt at trying to be tough. The point is: I just wasn't myself anymore.

My mom calls this period in my life "the dark years." It was the only time my mom and I ever went two weeks without speaking to each other, which is not something we do. She is my rock, and no matter where I am, we talk every day, if not multiple times a day.

But she wouldn't accept Angelo. He came home with me to Georgia for my birthday, and the problems started when I wanted him to see home videos of me when I was a little girl. He fell asleep, and my mom gave me a look. Then my mom made her gravy, the special gravy handed down from her mother and grandmother. I'd been talking this gravy up to him the entire trip. This was my family dish.

After dinner I asked him, "What did you think?"

"To be honest," he said, "it was a little bland."

Bland? I should have left him there and then, but of course I didn't.

The rest of the trip didn't go any better. My mother looked at Angelo as if he were a bug that needed to be squished. He was the opposite of everything she wanted for me. "I don't care at all what you say to me," she said point-blank. "He's a bad guy. He is killing your fire. I don't even recognize you anymore."

I knew things were bad when he started trying to take credit for songs he wasn't even in the room for. I remember asking him if I could have coproduction on a song I had helped create with a step-routine sound I did in high school, and he laughed at me. He was selfish. I think he was my boyfriend only to help further his career, which it did. He met many people through working with me that contributed to his connections and success today. Not to say he isn't talented, because he most certainly is, but there was a history of him dating or sleeping with people in the industry to position himself further along in his career. What I'm saying is he never really loved me or even liked me, now that I think about it. He couldn't possibly have with the way he treated me. He saw an opportunity and he took it.

My mom wasn't the only one who didn't approve of Angelo. Hallie—

surefire signs you have a terrible boyfriend

* He doesn't like it when you hang out with your friends or family.
* You lose touch with your friends and family.
* He makes you pay for everything (e.g., dinners on your birthday).
* After spending time with him, you feel worse about yourself, not better.
* Your personality changes—and not in a good way.
* He doesn't like your mom's cooking!

who ended up leaving Big Yellow Dog once I got a record deal to go around with me like a tour manager (but in her case, more like a big sister)—hated him. She was in constant communication with my mom. They would get on the phone and commiserate.

"We've got to get her out of this," my mom cried.

"I'm trying, Karen," Hallie said. "I can't get her away from him."

I stayed with Angelo because I felt very alone. But the more I stayed with him, the lonelier I felt. Of course, in the moment, I didn't see things that way. I didn't see anything. I was pushing forward, blinded by my own pain.

That's how I wound up in California, living with Angelo on the edge of Calabasas and Malibu. My family had moved from Georgia to Hawaii, Hallie was in Nashville, and I was in the hills of Los Angeles where I didn't know a single soul. When Angelo went away on trips, I was so pathetic that I would go stay at his place with his mom (yes,

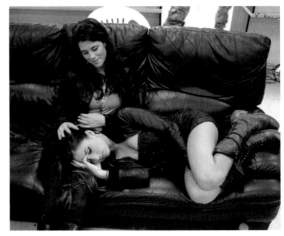

he still lived at home). I didn't want to be all by myself in my rental. Disconnected from everything and everyone, I became depressed.

About nine months after moving to Malibu, I found myself at LAX waiting for a flight back to Nashville for work. I was crying because my relationship with Angelo was over. There had been no big fight or revelation. Instead, it had been a quiet moment the night before.

We were in a hotel room on Sunset Boulevard, so I could be closer to the airport for my early flight the following day. Lying in bed, watching him, it felt like I could finally see clearly. When Angelo

don't ignore your gut

I always say those little knots you get in your stomach are there for a reason. I had those knots all the time with Angelo.

Listen to yourself! People are so much more intuitive than they think they are. If you get those knots in your stomach, or the hair on the back of your neck sticks up, or whatever little signal is trying to tell you "This isn't right," don't force it. It is *not* right.

If you won't listen to yourself, then listen to the people whom you love and trust. If they're telling you a relationship isn't good, you really should listen to them. Don't pull the us-against-the-world card, because you'll end up alone. Friends or family who have proven their love for you over time don't want to see you unhappy.

My relationship with Angelo created a wedge between my family and me that had never existed before. My sister and I were fighting over this. My mama and I didn't talk for a while. That red flag was so big it could have been seen from space.

It's no more complicated than this: if you don't feel good about yourself when you're with a guy, get rid of him.

looked at me, it was as though I was invisible and he could see right through me to the other side of the room. He didn't see me.

By this point we had dated for years, during which I was like that little girl in high school who wanted to be loved and accepted so badly.

No matter how much he hurt me, I kept fighting for our relationship and hoping he would love me. But I don't think he ever really loved me. In that moment in that hotel room, I finally could see that, and suddenly I was done. I felt nothing anymore.

From the airport, I emailed Angelo to break up with him. I didn't do it over the phone because I knew he would talk me out of it. "This isn't going to work," I wrote, and then closed my laptop.

Sitting at the gate, waiting for my flight to Nashville, all I wanted was my mama. That's when I looked up and saw a flight to Honolulu at another gate right by me. "What if I flew home right now?" I thought.

Since Steve flew for Delta so long, we still had some privileges (and I never traveled with anything more than a carry-on). I called my mom to see if there was any availability on the flight. "There is! There is!" she said. "I'll put you on it right now."

And so I blew off Nashville and got on the plane to Honolulu.

As soon as the flight took off, I started crying again. I was relieved to know I'd see my mama soon, but the terrible loneliness that had been with me for the last three years started to creep back in. I knew the relationship with Angelo was over, but I didn't know what was next.

Tired of feeling like a victim, I took out my laptop and started writing a letter directly to God about what I wanted more than anything else: a soul mate.

"I'm on the way to Hawaii to see my family," I wrote. "It's going to be my birthday soon. It would be the greatest gift to find my soul mate. I don't want to spend one more day without him."

My mom always said that when you're talking to God, be as descriptive as possible, because he's listening. So I got real specific.

Dear God,

Please send me my soul mate.

He has dark eyes and hair, and strong legs like a soccer player's.
I bet he's an athlete.

He makes the breakfast while I make the coffee.
I love his dog.

He makes me smile every day and doesn't judge me.

Then all of a sudden, in the middle of writing this letter, I started to feel real happiness, because I could feel him. I could feel my soul mate.

"He's out there," I thought. "He's there right now, somewhere in this world."

I probably sound like a nutjob, but I just felt it so strongly—this person existed. My prayers were going to be answered. I started crying on the plane again, but this time they were tears of joy.

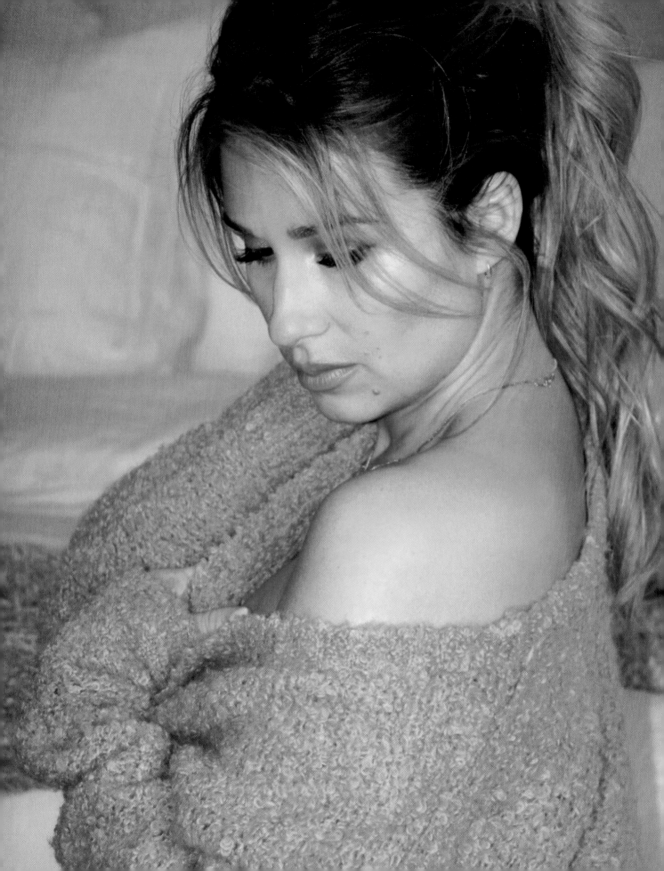

soul mate, where are you?

After I broke up with Angelo, I dated many, many guys. Like snowflakes, no two were alike.

There was the bartender, who was really easygoing and sweet. It was a nice change of pace from my previous experience, where nothing I did seemed right. This guy was a total one-eighty from Angelo. Six-foot-five and covered in tattoos, he had two pit bulls and two roommates who filled their little shack up with smoke (the roommates, not the dogs—poor things). But he thought I hung the moon, something I wasn't used to, and that was nice for a while. Nine months, to be precise.

Bartender Boy had no money. I mean none. He didn't have a car or a single cent to his name. He was broke the whole time we were together, so I paid for everything (not to mention drove him around). It's not like money is so important to me. Because I always made my own money, I was never the type of girl who thought, "I need to go find a rich husband." But Bartender Boy also lacked any kind of ambition. Yes, he was really fun and down for anything, but he also couldn't *afford* anything. Because he had no real plans, I tried everything to help him find a career, including suggesting he join the military (a few past criminal records kept him from that).

After the novelty of someone being nice to me wore off, I decided I should probably find someone who could pay for dinner once in a while—or at least be able to drive to dinner. Yet again I went in a wildly different direction. This time I went out with a former professional football player who was very financially solvent. Football Man, however, turned out to be even more short-lived than Bartender Boy. Our relationship came to an abrupt halt after we went out to dinner with a group of his friends. While I was telling a story about something probably really out there (since I have no real filter), he kicked me under the table and gave me a look. After we left the restaurant, he told me that I had embarrassed him.

I don't know about you, but I want a man who winks at me, even if I say something crazy, not kicks me. And I never want anyone to tell me that I'm embarrassing.

I dated many more guys after that, always looking for my perfect mate. I went out with one of the biggest baseball players of our generation but found him to be too vanilla—kind and sweet, but not enough for me. I also found myself going back and forth in my mind on one of my first loves, a country singer in Nashville, who I always thought would come back around but for some reason also never felt like the right fit.

I was searching. I wanted to find my soul mate so desperately, not to make me feel fulfilled—I was always confident in myself without a man— but because I wanted him, because I felt him close by and knew it was only

break up but don't break down

Everyone's allowed to be sad for a little bit. No matter how bad a relationship is, you've gotta mourn. It's only human.

Indulge your grief. Run yourself a bubble bath; have that glass of wine or champagne; put on a good breakup playlist. It's okay to have a good cry. But then get over it. You can't dwell on your sadness too long or it'll consume you.

Set goals and meet them. It can be anything from signing up at the gym (and actually going) to finally volunteering at a local animal shelter. Do something for yourself or others. This will not only help your self-esteem, but it'll distract you so that you can move on quicker.

I don't subscribe to the philosophy that you have to wait a long time before starting a new relationship after a failed one. I don't believe any of that. Cut your losses and start dating other people. That doesn't mean you need to go sleep with a bunch of people. I don't believe in that either. But you should start getting out there again and spend time with your friends. Don't hole up alone for too long.

If you were cheated on, get pissed and get into the best shape of your life to show that ex what you're made of!

Go to the gym. Go dancing or to the movies with your girlfriends. And start dating other people!

a matter of time until he and I would be together. I was missing my soul mate so dearly even though I didn't know him yet.

Every single guy I went out with during this period had a quality I was looking for, but I was really trying to find that perfect person. And none of them even came close. Still, each relationship taught me a lesson and helped to mold me. One even helped me find the woman who'd become my makeup artist, stylist, and best friend.

I was seeing a rocker guy, whom we'll just call Cuckoo Bird since it's a pretty accurate name. We were staying at a hotel after a show of his in Texas. I was lounging in the hotel room while he went out for a bit to grab some cigarettes (no, this relationship was not one of my finest moments) when the phone rang. I answered, and on the other end was the voice of an angel. Seriously, she was the sweetest-sounding person I'd ever heard— and she was looking for Cuckoo.

"Who's this?" I asked.

"I'm his fiancée," said the woman on the phone.

"He's engaged?"

"Yes."

"There's no way! He said that he was single."

I had no idea. I'm never *that* girl. There are plenty of men out there. I didn't have to date married ones or engaged ones.

"I'm looking at my wedding dress," she said.

My heart sank, because I knew instinctively that she was telling the truth. She went on to tell me that this had happened multiple times before and that she wasn't angry with me, since she was sure I had no clue, but that she really needed to speak with her fiancé.

At that moment, Cuckoo Bird walked back into the hotel room, and I hung up on her without thinking.

"You're engaged? Your fiancée just called!" I yelled at him.

We started in on a big old fight that ended with him passing out asleep (men can do that kind of thing; it's amazing). I threw my stuff in my bag, went downstairs, got a taxi, headed to the airport, and never talked to him again.

But I did hear from his fiancée. Out of the blue, she reached out months later after she had forgiven him and married him. I didn't know if it was closure or curiosity, but Jessica—as I learned her name was—and I wound up talking on the phone for three hours. And it had nothing to do with Cuckoo Bird. We talked about our careers (she's a makeup artist) and growing up in small southern towns (she's from Tennessee). We hit it off so well, she wanted to meet up. I wasn't so sure about that, and neither

was Hallie. It seemed kind of weird. What if our entire phone conversation was an act, and she was looking for some kind of revenge?

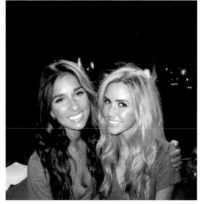

In the end, faith in humanity won over fear, and I decided to meet Jessica in person. Like a friendship fairy tale, I fell madly in love with her. She had such great style and taste. We shared more than a love of makeup and cool clothes—we were small-town girls with big dreams.

Fast-forward, Jessica and I have been best friends for more than ten years. Since we met, her career has completely taken off. I had her style me early on, and she has been my stylist and makeup artist ever since. And I'm really particular about my makeup. I won't let anyone else touch my face but Jessica. If she's unavailable, I do it myself. So if you ever see my makeup looking great on the red carpet or TV, it's only one of the two of us.

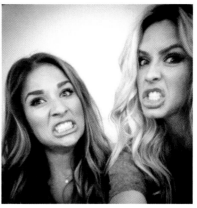

We always joke that the one thing Cuckoo had going for him is his great taste in women, because "we are fabulous," as we say.

Seriously, though, Jessica and I are grateful Cuckoo was a slimeball; otherwise we would never have met. We always say the reason this terrible man entered both of our lives was so we could meet. We need each other. I need her in my life. She's not only my best friend but has her own relationship with my mom and my sister. Jessica calls my mother all the time. She and Sydney take their own girls' trips. She's *our* best friend. Or really part of our family. We say that if Mom and Steve had a baby girl, it would have been Jessica.

But first we had to get rid of Cuckoo Bird. But that wasn't until much later. We both still had a lot of heartache to endure until we each found our Prince Charming. After she finally dumped Cuckoo, to make up for, well, dating her fiancé, I introduced her to Logan, one of Eric's college teammates. (They got married, and Jessica is now living her own fairy tale. She's the happiest she's ever been in her life.)

I went through a lot of wrong guys until I experienced something I'd never thought would happen to me.

Rock bottom.

I was at the end of my record deal in Nashville and was on the verge of depression. I felt like my music career was at a standstill with no real future plans. My judgment was off, and my family was far away. I was going out with friends every night, but I was lonelier and more vulnerable than I had ever been before.

Although I went out with a bunch of men, I didn't sleep around. I didn't like guys thinking that they were special enough to have that from me, so I was very protective of myself. I let my guard down with one guy after dating him for a few months, however—and then I didn't hear from him again! I had heard those stories from friends about jerks who disappeared once they got what they wanted, but that didn't happen to me. The guys I chose to share time with, though they might not have been the most amazing guys, at least always called. I had never felt so violated and disappointed in myself. "Who have I become?" I asked myself.

After three days of not hearing from him and beating myself up for that mistake, I actually called the guy and chewed him out. I told him he would never get over me and would regret this and that he was a man-child. It was a rookie move, sure. But I was so pissed off that I had let someone like him get the better of me. After that, I took my own advice and decided I had done enough wallowing. I was also done with dating. "Guys suck," I determined. "I'm going to focus on me and my career. I am just done."

BLISSED OUT

The right man should give you confidence, bring out the best in you, and make you feel amazing. You should feel bliss.

It's ridiculous to say you're going to feel bliss 100 percent of the time, but 95 percent of the time is totally reasonable. I have it in my marriage 95 percent of the time. The other 5 percent has nothing to do with either one of us; it's just real life. But I'm happy every day, all day—because I love my husband and am content in my marriage. That's how it should be.

Everyone deserves that. I don't like when people sell themselves short by saying, "Not everyone gets a fairy tale." Why not? You do deserve a fairy tale, and don't let anyone tell you otherwise.

I've experienced firsthand the bad and the good in relationships. Time and time again, I've witnessed the remarkable transformation from the loneliness of being with the wrong person to the satisfaction of being madly in love with a soul mate. Fundamentally, "settling" is never worth it and always ends in misery. You get one life, so you might as well pick the right partner to spend it with.

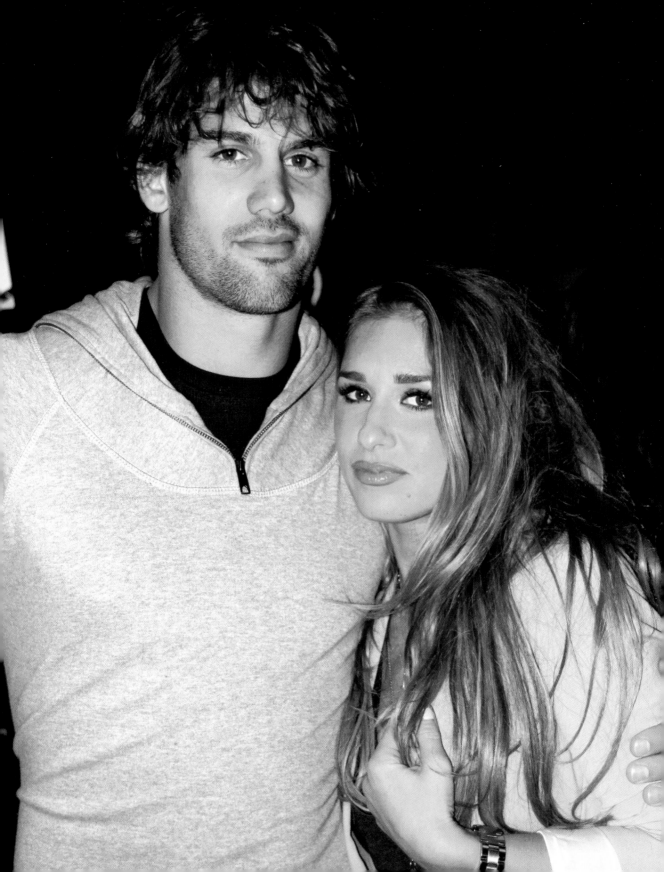

completion

Twenty-four hours after chewing out the one and only guy who ghosted me after I let my guard down and feeling as if I had hit rock bottom, I pulled myself together. After a dose of self-loathing, I put my big-girl panties on. I had a show in Jacksonville, Florida, the following day, which couldn't have been better timing. I needed the distraction of work, and hanging with my band always cheered me up. We were all out eating when I got a text message from a friend named Liana, who was all about matchmaking. She knew I was single and had me on her mind any time an eligible bachelor came around. She was in Arizona hanging with a guy she had been seeing, and that guy was rooming with my Eric.

"I'm sitting at dinner with one of the hottest guys I've ever seen," she texted me. "If I wasn't dating his friend, I'd be all over this guy. His name is Eric Decker. He's a football player."

Ugh. I had dated a football player, and it didn't go well. I had dated a lot of guys, and none of it had gone well.

I texted back, "I am swearing off men right now."

My friend texted a picture of him she took while he was barely paying attention. I can still remember that picture. Dressed in blue jeans and a white T-shirt, he was sitting with his legs crossed in a relaxed pose with those dark eyes and dark hair and cinnamon-colored skin. My mouth hit the ground; he was beautiful.

"He's stunning but y'all are in Arizona," I texted.

Liana refused to give up and began to play matchmaker back in Arizona. She showed him pictures of me, and he apparently was familiar with who I was from my song "I Look So Good (Without You)," because it had been a hit in his home state of Minnesota. He asked my friend for my number and texted me right away.

THE CHASE

I had made way too many mistakes in my dating career. Starting from the very first text from Eric, I decided I would do things differently this time around. From now on, if a man wanted me, he was going to have to show it. So I made Eric chase me. He was going to have to do all the work to prove he wanted me.

I wouldn't call it game playing. I'd call it common sense. Women should always have the upper hand in the early stages of a relationship, in my opinion. You've got to be busy, because men like the chase. They are like hungry tigers on the hunt.

I made Eric hunt for me. Even though I was so excited after our first phone conversation that I emailed my mom photos and an interview with him that I had found online, he would never have known it. I never texted, called, or anything-ed him first. I'm not kidding. For the first three months of our relationship, he never got an incoming call from me.

Once Eric decided he wasn't going to text me all day, because he was tired of always being the one to take the initiative.

Did I call him?

Nope.

I didn't hear from him until the middle of the next day, when he gave in and called. "I was just testing to see if you would call me," he said. "Why am I always the one reaching out?"

Because you're going to have to work for me.

I didn't say it out loud, but that was my mind-set—not only because I had been burned in the past, but also because Eric was a good-looking football player used to girls fawning all over him. Eric didn't disappoint. He worked very hard to try to get me.

After talking on the phone, texting, and video-chatting for a good four weeks, he asked to meet me. That'd be fine, but again, he was going to have to take the initiative. If he wanted to see me, he could plan a trip.

Although as a wide receiver for the Broncos he was based out of Denver, Eric was living in Minnesota for the summer. He got a flight from the Midwest to Nashville to spend the weekend with me.

I'll never forget the first time our eyes met—in person. I had been at the studio all day. The session ran overtime, so I had to make some last-minute logistical changes that included my girlfriend and roommate dropping off my mom (who had been visiting me) at the airport and picking up Eric (who still claims to this day that that was rude). Maybe it wasn't all about my studio session

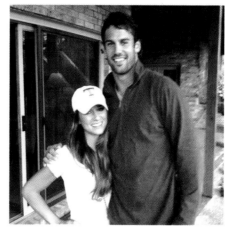

First photo of us on the second day we spent together.

going long. I was so nervous I wanted my
roommate to feel him out for me. My mom
was actually the one to have the first look.
As she headed to her gate, she walked past
Eric while he was coming off the plane. She
stopped to introduce herself, then texted me
this one little thought: "He's stunning. Try
not to sleep with him."

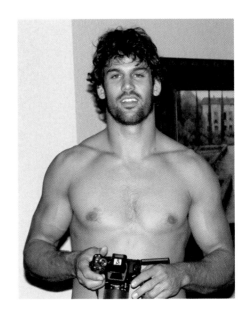

After she picked Eric up, my roommate
dropped him at Kalamatas, a Mediterranean
restaurant that I loved. My producer dropped
me off. Eric would tell me that, upon seeing
me get out of the car through the restaurant
window, I was even tinier than he had thought. I walked in the door to
find this man: pair of blue jeans and a white tee, with a little bit of sweat
around his stunning face from being so nervous. He stood up and was even
bigger than I had imagined. I hugged him hello and felt his strong body
and arms wrap around me. I was in trouble.

I knew Eric was good-looking before I met him. The bigger surprise
was how he could just *be*. He was comfortable. Not to say that he wasn't
nervous, because he definitely was—and shy. He later told me that in the
beginning he was intimidated by me, big-time. "I was scared of you for the
first year," he said, "because you were just so intense. Your personality is so
strong."

Despite that, Eric looked at me in a different way than any other man
had before. He stared at me with his own form of quiet, calm intensity. It
wasn't a "Ooh, she's hot" ogling. I'd seen that plenty of times in the past.
The way he looked at me, I could tell that he was really taking me in (I
never caught him looking at anything but my eyes), and that made me feel
so confident while I was around him.

I guess the feeling was mutual, because before Eric left to return to Minnesota after our three-day weekend, he asked if we could be exclusive—and I said yes.

THE FAIRY TALE (WITH A FEW NECESSARY TWEAKS)

Eric kept coming at me. He called, texted, visited, everything. I could feel his love, devotion, and respect, but he didn't know how to court me. Before we met, he had been in only one relationship—his high school girlfriend, whom he dated for seven years. They were babies when they met, so Eric had no idea what it meant to date as an adult. Basically, he was raised to go dutch.

The first time we went out to dinner, I pulled out my credit card at the end—just for show—and he gave it to the waiter along with his card! I

ERIC SAYS

What initially attracted me to Jess—apart from her obvious good looks—was her sense of humor and how easy it was to have a conversation with her. We got deep, soon. For me that was big, because I'm a pretty reserved person. Jess brought me out of my shell, which I knew was going to be good for me. Plus, she was career-driven and a go-getter, qualities I wanted in a woman. However, it might have been her cooking that sealed the deal. The first time I visited her in Nashville, she cooked jambalaya. And I'm from Minnesota, where there's not a lot of spicy or ethnic-type food. And I fell in love. It's true: the way to a man's heart is through his stomach. At least this man. I love food. That's how she hooked me.

guess we were splitting the bill. I was so shocked that I didn't even think to protest. We went out a few more times, and the same thing happened again and again. He never offered to cover the bill or flights when I came in to visit him. Honestly, I thought maybe he was broke because of how frugal he was, so much so that I offered to cover his gas money when he picked me up from the airport.

Then I snapped out of it. He was an NFL player; he wasn't broke. Finally I decided, "Hell, no. I'm not doing this again."

It wasn't a matter of money, and it had nothing to do with being a bad guy; Eric does the right thing all the time. He was just clueless. Clueless.

"Look, I'm from the South," I explained. "In the South, the men pay for the movies, and they pay for the dinners. I'll get the coffees here and there, but you've got to step it up."

(When my brother was a freshman in high school, he was in a panic over having enough cash from my parents to take a date out to the movies and for popcorn.)

Eric was so embarrassed, and we never went dutch again. I tell this story not to embarrass my hubby, who is the most generous man in the world, but to say that even the most wonderful fairy-tale romance takes a little work. You can't throw in the towel at the first sign of imperfection. I knew Eric was a great guy; he just needed a little help. Like I needed some help (and trust me, I needed help too). We learned a lot from each other. So patience is an important aspect of dating (but not too much patience, if you know what I mean).

It's ironic that I'm talking about patience considering the fact that from the moment Eric and I met, our relationship moved really fast. Part of it was how right things felt between us, and part of it was timing.

Before meeting Eric, I had already decided I was done with Nashville. I needed a break. All the people important to me there had moved, including

Hallie, who went to New York. Plus, my lease was up—and my career was slowing down.

It's not easy making money in the music industry. Even when you get a big paycheck, the percentage taken out by all the people on an artist's team is also big. Right off the bat, 15 to 20 percent goes to a manager. Then another 5 percent to a business manager. An additional 10 to 15 percent goes to an agent. In all, that can total nearly 50 percent of your income. Then throw in taxes.

Yes, I was given six figures from my label for my first record deal, which is a ton of money. But after I paid all those percentages and the taxes, I was left with about $20,000 to pay for my car, rent, food, and travel for two years. That went pretty quickly.

I got out of my lease and moved back in with my parents, where I hoped to be for no more than a month. My next move was going to be to LA to live with Jessica, who was getting a divorce from Cuckoo Bird. She was looking for an apartment—and a job for me at the makeup place where she worked, so I would have a source of income while I continued to make music.

When I told Eric about my plans to move to California, he said, "No, you're not. Come to Denver."

His asking me to move in with him came out of nowhere. First of all, we had been dating for only a few months, and we definitely never had a conversation about living together. It was a shock for everyone, including Eric, who had never taken that step with his previous girlfriend. But Eric said he was afraid he was going to lose me out there.

The hardest part of my decision was delivering the news to Jessica. "I'm so sorry," I told her, "but he wants me to move to Denver, and my heart's telling me I should."

So I did.

dating dos and don'ts

Now you can say all this is silly and game playing, but I landed my man. So in the words of Forrest Gump, "That's all I have to say about that."

DON'T CALL OR TEXT A GUY FIRST.
I know some women say they don't like to play games, but this worked for me—and all my friends who took my advice. Men like the chase!

DO BE A BUSY GIRL.
When a guy asks what you're doing, never say "Nothing." Always appear to be busy. It's more appealing.

DON'T ALWAYS TEXT BACK IMMEDIATELY.
Make him work for you and wonder what you're doing during those long periods of silence.

DON'T SEND TEXTS THAT ARE LONGER THAN A SENTENCE.
Do not send men paragraphs. This isn't a book. They don't want to read your stories and emotional journeys. Men get so drained from that, they just turn off their phones. Guys don't want too much information, so get to the point.

DON'T GOSSIP ABOUT FRIENDS OR EXES.
They don't care.

DO ASK HIM ABOUT HIS CHILDHOOD.
Men love talking about themselves (even if they pretend like they don't). Learning personal information about them also makes them a little vulnerable, which can give you an upper hand.

DON'T SLEEP WITH A GUY ON THE FIRST DATE.
It gives the wrong idea. Make him earn it.

DO SMILE.
Always have a bubbly, happy energy. Men want to be around someone who makes them feel happy and at ease. A Debbie Downer will make them wish they could bail and hang with their friends. You want to be so cool that they would rather hang with you than them any day.

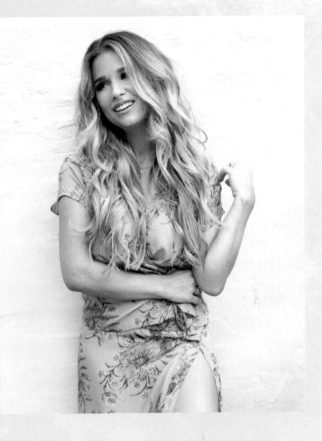

DON'T PRETEND YOU LEFT SOMETHING OVER AT HIS PLACE JUST TO GET HIM TO TEXT YOU. Guys see right through those kinds of tricks, which only come off as desperate.

DON'T JUMP TO ANGER RIGHT AWAY.
Instead of getting all fired up, take twenty minutes to cool off. Sit back and think about the situation from a different angle. (This is advice from my mama, who is like my counselor so I don't have to pay someone.)

DO LOOK YOUR BEST BUT NOT OVER THE TOP.
Put in effort without him knowing you put in any effort. You don't want to be so made up that you freak him out when he finally sees you with no tan, makeup, false lashes, nails, etc.

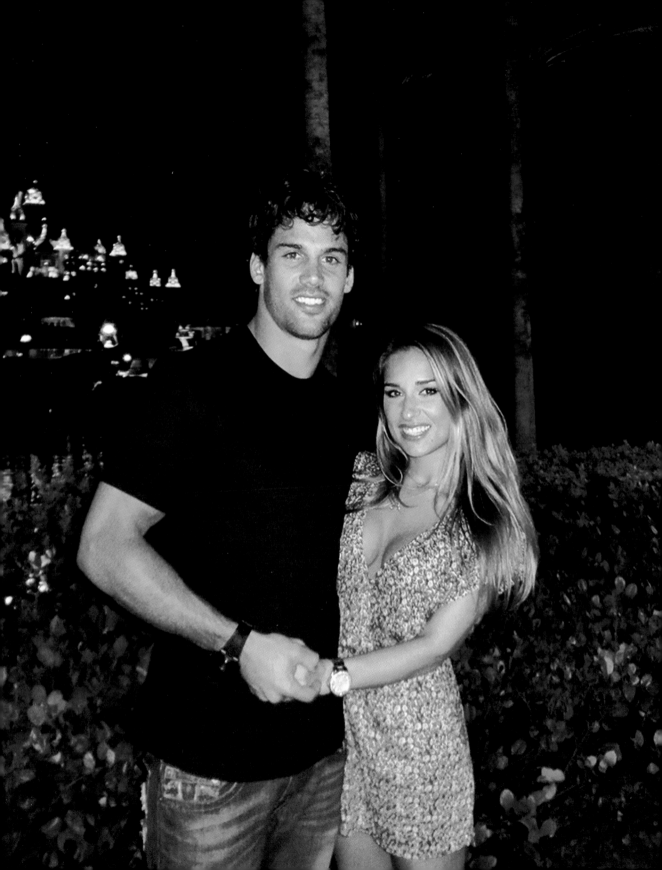

reality check

Eric and I had been dating three months when he asked me to move to Colorado. I know it sounds crazy since we had only known each other for such a short while, but it couldn't have come at a better time. I needed to begin a new chapter, which before meeting Eric had originally been to move in with Jess in LA and work part-time doing makeup while trying to get another record deal. But Eric wasn't having it. He wanted my new chapter to be with him full-time in Colorado.

I followed my heart, but moving to Denver was a risk, both personally and professionally. I was ostensibly putting my career on a huge hold when I accepted Eric's offer.

The decision was made a little easier by the fact that my music career wasn't going all that great. I'd lost my record deal in a process that, although it was mutual, was also long, slow, and painful. I never liked how the label tried to market me or the songs it chose to push. So when I went on a radio tour to promote myself to stations throughout the country, I had a really hard time. It's never easy to ask people to like you (in this case, program directors and on-air personalities), but it's pretty much impossible to convince radio stations when you don't like what the label has done with you or your music either. No surprise, the radio stations didn't play me, and if you didn't have radio back then, you had nothing. (Thank God, now it's different. Social media and television have changed everything. Here's proof: in 2017, I had a number one album on *Billboard*'s US Top Country Albums chart without any airtime.)

My label didn't officially drop me, but it shelved me—which was just a more polite version of the same thing. It didn't think there was a place for me anymore in its stable of musicians, so I asked to be let out of my contract, and it complied.

The rational thing to do would have been for me to stay in Nashville or move to LA to write more music and try to get a new deal. But through this dark phase, Eric was such a light in my life. My heart was pulled toward him, no matter what it meant for my career.

Everything slowed down for the next two years, because I didn't have a record deal and wasn't actively writing and recording. But it was so worth it. On your deathbed, are you going to think, "I had such a great career"? Or are you going to say, "Man, my family really loved me." I really think everything happens for a reason. If I had been crazy busy trying to juggle a huge career, I wouldn't have been able to foster my relationship with Eric and create such a strong foundation. During those early years, we were attached at the hip, and I loved every minute of it.

Those were also some of the happiest years of my life. I loved Colorado—spending every morning in our robes drinking coffee, gazing at the snow-covered mountains, and playing with our golden puppies. It was just amazing.

Not long after I arrived in Denver, Sydney moved in with us! Now, I know for a lot of folks having your little sister come live with you and your new boyfriend would be a nightmare. But not Sydney. I couldn't have been given a better sister. For starters, she doesn't have a jealous bone in her body. Even though I've been in the spotlight our entire lives, she has never, not once, been envious or angry about it. Never. The opposite: she has always been happy for me. Maybe because we look out for each other. Through all my successes, I keep her right there with me. She's along for the ride. Anything I have, I give to her too; I want to share with her without her ever having to ask.

A perfect example is when Sydney was having a hard time in school. She went to college for two years to pursue a degree in education because she wanted to be a schoolteacher. College, however, wasn't for her. Struggling with her courses and the party scene (which is just not our thing), she was very unhappy. Lost, she didn't know what to do next. She wanted to leave school, but my parents weren't for that. She gave me a call, crying about how hard it was: she couldn't handle it anymore. I told her (against my parents' wishes), "Just drop out and come live with me."

And for three years, she did.

Eric loved having Sydney there just as much as I did. That's one of the reasons I fell in love with him. He fit in with my family right from the start. After we had been dating only a month, I told him casually on the phone about my dad being promoted to colonel and how we were all getting together to celebrate that coming weekend in San Antonio. He invited himself to come instantly, which threw me off. But my mom reassured me that his wanting to meet my family so soon and be a part of the celebration was a great quality. He joined us, and I have to say this was the moment I knew I loved him. He fit right in as if we had been together for years. He went golfing with my dad, wrestled with my brother, and teased my little sister. He instantly loved my mama too and

I didn't need any convincing that Eric was a good man, but I'm happy that one of the first things we did together as a couple was get a dog. That's one of my best pieces of advice to women—if you can, get a dog with your guy before you have children. It'll tell you so much about if he really is a caretaker.

Eric and I got two dogs! Jake and Jenny. Jake is Eric's dog. They have a special relationship. Eric isn't always the best at using his words. He's a man. After a hard game or other letdown, he doesn't want to talk about his feelings. All he wants to do is pet Jake, who nuzzles up and makes him feel better. We call Jake his healer, or now, since we started our foundation, his emotional service dog. Jake was the inspiration for Deckers Dogs, which rescues dogs from kill shelters, trains them to become emotional support animals, and sends them home with veterans suffering from post-traumatic stress disorder. We all know how hard coming home can be, not just on the men and women who have sacrificed so much for our country and freedoms, but on their families as well. These dogs, able to sense when their owner feels threatened, provide a lot of comfort and reassurance (including going into homes first and turning on all the lights!).

It was Jenny (who would become my daughter Vivi's dog) who taught me that Eric was way more than just a great boyfriend. Soon after we got our second golden retriever, she was sick and throwing up all over the house. Eric didn't lose his temper or even leave me to deal with the situation. Instead, he sat there patiently rubbing Jenny's back and telling her to "Let it out. Let it out. You're okay." In that moment, when I saw his sweet, nurturing, and patient nature in action, I realized that Eric was going to be a wonderful daddy someday.

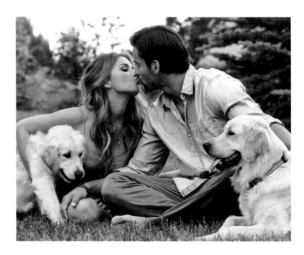

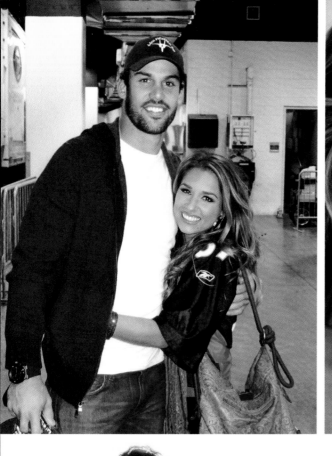
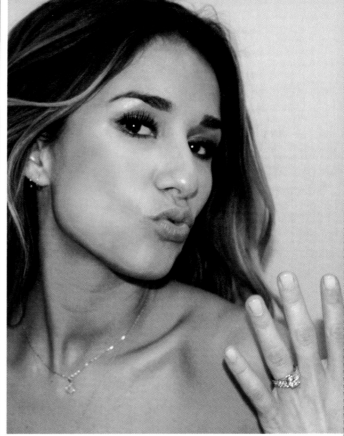
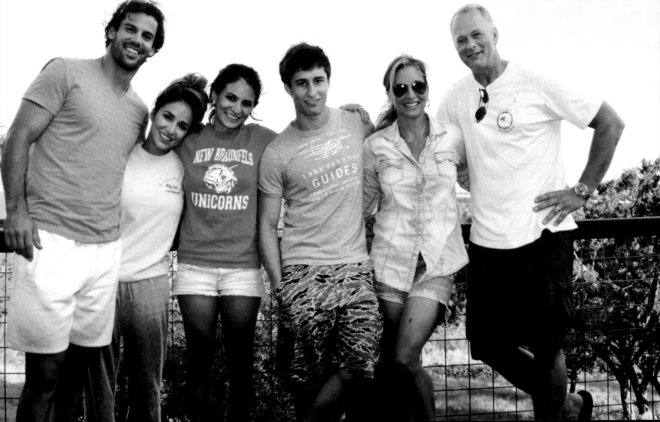

NOT-SO-PERFECT PROPOSAL

I wanted to propose to Jess on our one-year anniversary, which coincided with the Academy of Country Music Awards in Las Vegas. I had bought the ring and flew out to Vegas to meet her. When I checked into our hotel, I asked for the manager. Because breakfast with coffee has always kind of been our thing, I wanted to ask her to marry me while we had breakfast in bed. I explained to the manager that room service should place the ring in one of the dishes when I ordered breakfast the following morning. I pictured Jess pulling off a plate cover only to discover an engagement ring and me on one knee. Then I gave the manager the ring.

I was so nervous when room service pulled into the suite in the morning.

"We're good?" I asked the waiter knowingly.

"Yeah, we're good," he said.

But when we started lifting the silver covers keeping the plates warm, there was nothing but eggs, fruit, and pancakes.

What the—? Where was it?

I looked under the tablecloth covering the rolling tray. Nothing. I was no longer nervous, I was downright panicking. Someone had just stolen my ring, and I didn't have insurance on it yet!

I couldn't think straight. I wanted to call the manager, but I didn't want to ruin the surprise. Maybe I should just tell Jess what was going on?

Meanwhile, she could tell my head was somewhere else. "Why aren't you eating?" she asked, offering me a cup of coffee and a concerned expression. Oh great, now I had not only messed up this proposal but also made her worry.

A few minutes later (although it felt more like a few hours), there was a knock on the hotel door. It was the waiter. "Got it," he said, holding out the ring box.

"Where was this when I needed it?" I snapped.

Although I was relieved to have the very expensive ring back, I was still incredibly stressed out. Just then Jess called from the bedroom of our hotel suite: "What is it?"

I had to think fast. "Just a couple of waters!"

"Okay, bring them in here."

"Why don't you come get it?"

"What?"

"Just come here and get it."

"What's wrong with you?" she said, tying her robe as she walked into the living room. There she found me on my knee, ring in hand.

The proposal wasn't how I imagined it going down, but in a way it was very much us: messy and not always the way we planned. But it always works out for us.

saw where I got a lot of my personality. It might have been my jambalaya that sealed the deal for him, but for me it was watching him with my family.

Sydney, Eric, and I had so much fun. I would make dinner, and she would make dessert. It was a team effort. And we all would watch movies in the theater downstairs. We took care of one another just like we always have.

My home life was great, but I still struggled socially. Because of my experiences in school with bullying, I was awkward. Scratch that. I was phobic. As a pro football player, Eric had a lot of events and parties he needed to attend. Of course he assumed that I, as his girlfriend, would go with him. And I did. But I sat in the corner by myself, not talking to anyone, because I was in such a panic and sweating. Whenever Eric tried to beckon me over, I refused. It was awful.

It didn't take long for Eric to call me out on it. I think it was the third event we attended for a football function when he asked, "Why don't you come talk with me? I don't understand."

I explained to him that from my corner where I sat all alone, I could tell nobody in the room liked me. Eric was sweet, as he always is, but firm.

"You could not be more wrong. You need to give people a chance," he said. "We've got to get over this. Your place is right by my side, shaking hands and talking to people. This is important to me, and not just for my job. I need you to be my first lady."

Although I had so much anxiety, Eric helped me through the process of opening up. From then on, he would grab my hand at a party and hold it tight in order to make me stand there next to him. I was terrified, but feeling my hand in his big, strong one brought me a lot of comfort—and eventually confidence. It wasn't easy and took a lot of time, but I finally got over the idea that everyone hated me right off the bat. Now, Eric is the one who has to pull me away from chatting at events.

He just had a way about him that made me feel good. I'm an Aries, a fire sign, and Eric's a Pisces, which is a water sign. He and I do really well together. I have a lot of ideas and creativity, which means I can say the weirdest, craziest things sometimes. But Eric never judges me or thinks I'm weird. When I say something that is so bananas, all he says is, "That's what makes you special." And he means it; he is just so open-minded. I always said I needed to marry someone who loves me in the way my mother does—unconditionally and judgment-free, so that it doesn't kill that light in me. He makes me feel like I can do and say anything, and he will still be right by my side, smiling. I have so much confidence now in who I am. We both helped each other grow into the people we wanted to be.

So beyond his good looks, strong work ethic, and great dad potential, I knew he was the right man for me—because I felt like the right woman when I was with him.

GAME ON

As soon as we got engaged in 2012, we had a producer reach out to me through my Facebook page to see if we'd be interested in doing a reality show together on our journey to the altar.

I had always wanted to do a reality show, because I thought it would be a good way for the public to get to know the real me—and not the me that my previous label had put out there. Because my team got me exposure only in outlets like *Maxim* magazine (and I mean wearing-only-a-guitar kind of exposure), my female fan base was nonexistent. The only fans I ever had were men. I got fan mail from men in jail. It was bad. I kept telling the president of my label, "We should try to get me a reality show. I really think it would help with the music." The answer, though, was always no because of a bad experience in the past with one of his artists and a reality show.

This time, when I was approached about doing a show, it felt like the perfect opportunity not only to kick my music career back into gear the right way but also to tell our great love story. Why not take advantage of the opportunity to document such a special time in our lives? I knew Eric and I would cherish it forever.

Never mind that being engaged is often a stressful time for a couple, and I had a fiancé who, while supportive of me as an entertainer, definitely didn't dream of having cameras following him around.

Eric was nervous when I first brought the idea to him. He was used to performing on the field, but this was definitely out of his comfort zone.

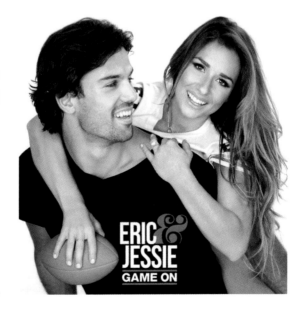

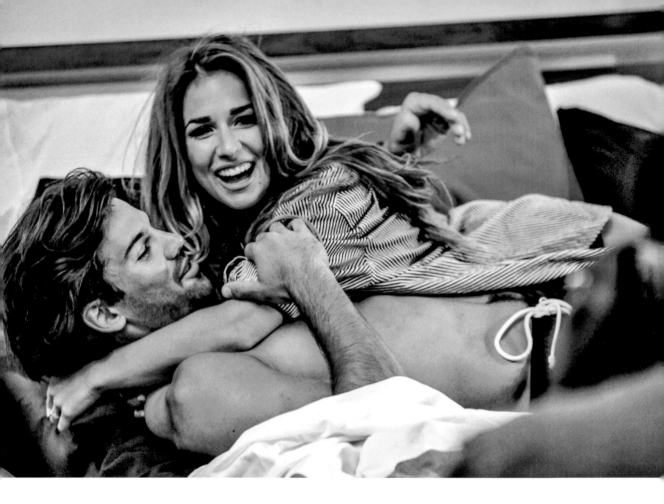

But I had no doubts everything would work out. "I will take the reins when it comes to this," I told him. "You won't have to worry about a thing. Let's just be open and honest. We don't need to try to put on a show. Let's just be exactly who we are."

He trusted me. In return I fought extremely hard to keep the final product as authentic as possible. Of course, TV folks want there to be drama, whether it's manufactured or real. Any time I saw things going the way of made up, the hair on the back of my neck went right up. It wasn't just my reputation on the line—I had also involved the man I loved. No one was going to mess with him.

At one point, two of the producers were trying to manipulate us with the questions—so I had them fired. I don't play when it comes to my family. It began when they were interviewing my sister. One of them asked her something so inappropriate that the cameraman looked at her from behind the producer and mouthed the words, "Don't answer that." Then during my interview, this producer tried to provoke me into acting jealous about my future husband's career!

"What's it like watching Eric's career take off when yours isn't doing anything?" he asked.

"When Eric's doing well, I'm doing well. Why wouldn't I want him to succeed?" I said.

"Come on," he went on. "It must be hard. Especially when he's in photo shoots with gorgeous models, you know . . ."

As soon as that happened, I marched my butt outside and knocked on the window of the production van parked outside our home. They rolled it down, and I let them have a piece of my mind.

"What is your point? What are you trying to do here?"

That wasn't the end. I called the head of the production company and said I wanted those producers off the project: "Or I'm not doing another day of this show."

I ended up getting my way. But my getting so upset over the show was the only thing that ever tried our relationship. The feeling that I always had to fight wore me out. Eric and I never had an argument about the show, and we never did anything we weren't comfortable with. He just didn't like to see me so stressed out. Any new experience, though, is a challenge. I wanted to make sure when our show hit the air it was as authentic and genuine to us as possible. And that's a lot of work.

Luckily, Paulina Williams, an incredible, brilliant producer, saved the day. Because I ended up trusting only her, she had to do the work of two producers! But she shared my vision. "This is good the way it is," she said. "This is why we chose you. I don't need to create anything."

I sure hoped so.

GAME REALLY ON

The night our show *Eric & Jessie: Game On* premiered on September 29, 2013, all those bad old high school feelings came flooding back. I thought I was going to puke, I felt so sick. I was afraid people were going to watch and instantly hate me. "Girls are going to judge me," I thought. "They're going to say I'm ugly and stupid and annoying." The negative voices in my head drowned out Eric and me on TV.

I decided to go on Twitter and search my name to see what people were saying, which was pretty much the worst idea in the world, because social media breeds a lot of haters. Except it wasn't.

I was shocked to find I had gained twenty thousand followers and that every single tweet was positive!

"I've never seen this girl before, but I like her!"

"I wanna be friends with her!!"

"OMG, I love Jessie!"

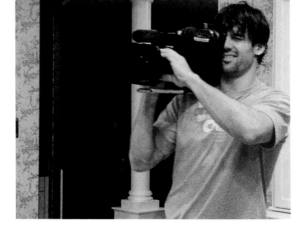

I couldn't believe that people were saying nice things about me. Actually, I couldn't believe that *women* were saying nice things about me. It was always my dream to have girls in my corner—and to be a role model to them. I was so happy that for the first time, through this show, they were not judging me at first glance but getting to know me.

From the first episode of *Eric & Jessie: Game On,* I gained so many female fans and followers. But the moment I truly experienced the shift in my fan base was when I did a meet and greet in Boston for the Macy's tree lighting. It was my first public appearance after the show's debut, because I took a lot of time off after the birth of my first child, Vivianne (more on that later in chapter 9).

When the publicity team told me about the event, I thought, "Why are they going to have me do a meet and greet? No one's going to stand in line to see me. It doesn't make any sense."

But when I got to the department store I was astonished by what I saw: a line out the door that wrapped around the building—of all girls. My mom was with me, and even as my biggest fan, she couldn't believe it either. Nothing like this had ever happened to me before.

Not long after, someone asked me to fill in for an artist who'd dropped out of a charity show at the Tin Roof, a Nashville bar and music venue. As part of a lineup of different singers, all I had to do was go on and sing five songs, but I hadn't played a show in years, ever since I lost my record deal. Still, I agreed. It was a great opportunity for me as a musician.

I tweeted and posted on Instagram about the show, not thinking that it'd have any real effect. When I was about to take the stage at the Tin Roof, however, there were probably six hundred girls all dressed like me in plaid shirts and bandannas.

"Are they all here to see me?" I asked the stage manager.

"Yes," he said.

It nearly made me cry how these beautiful girls sang all the words to my songs. Although it was happening right before my eyes, I couldn't believe it.

Fast-forward a few years later, and it's still happening. When I play sold-out venues for thousands of people, they're all girls, dressed just like me. (While I ditched the vixen image, I still wear sexy outfits. It's just that the personality to go with them is now more funny/goofy. You get a good body only once. I don't want to be an old lady regretting, "I shoulda worn those cutoff shorts when I had the chance.") There are maybe three or four men tops in the crowd (brought there by their daughters, wives, or girlfriends); otherwise it's women, singing to the music right alongside me. When I look out at my audience, I feel a tremendous sense

my faves

When I'm on tour or at meet and greets, my fans are always asking me about the things I like—movies, music, food, you name it. Here's my ultimate love list:

MY FAVORITE MOVIES

Forrest Gump: I connect with this movie on so many levels, from the music to the southern roots to the era it's set in. (I swear I was reincarnated from the '60s.) I love it so much I named my son Forrest.

My Cousin Vinny: This is the plane movie for Eric and me. Anytime we have a major flight I pull out my laptop and the dual connector for earphones. I hit play, and we both smile and laugh throughout the entire thing as if we've never seen it.

Vicky Cristina Barcelona: Penélope Cruz is my favorite actress, and I love that her husband, Javier Bardem, is in the movie as well. They're one of my favorite Hollywood couples. This movie is so beautiful and filled with dark humor.

Walk the Line: No matter how much I watch this movie, I'm always inspired by it. Reese Witherspoon is so infectious, and of course it's set in my favorite era: the '60s.

Selena: I love how close Selena Quintanilla was with her family and how supportive they were of her dream (it reminds me of my family)—and, of course, she had incredible presence.

Son in Law: My siblings and I could watch this over and over again. It turned me into a huge Pauly Shore fan.

It's Complicated: I love everything about this movie—the main character's stunning home, the food she makes. I think this is one of Meryl Streep's best, and Alec Baldwin is hilarious.

MY FAVORITE TV SHOWS

Friends
Sex and the City
Schitt's Creek
Impractical Jokers

(SOME OF) MY FAVORITE ALBUMS

Miranda Lambert, *Kerosene*
Lana Del Rey, *Born to Die*
Shelby Lynne, *Just a Little Lovin'*
Nickelback, *All the Right Reasons*
Forrest Gump soundtrack
Christina Aguilera, *Stripped*
Kacey Musgraves, *Same Trailer Different Park*
Sam Hunt, *Montevallo*
Shania Twain, *Come on Over*

FAVE ACTRESSES
Penélope Cruz
Reese Witherspoon
Jennifer Aniston
Goldie Hawn

FAVE COLORS
Pink
Baby blue

FAVE RESTAURANTS
Tommy Bahama and Quality Meats
in New York City

FAVE DRINK
Red wine

FAVE BEVERAGE
Unsweetened mango or tropical
iced tea

FAVE VACATION SPOT
Cabo San Lucas

FAVE FOODS
Cajun
Seafood

FAVE DESSERTS
Chocolate chip cookies
Chocolate ganache cake

FAVE CANDLE
Paddywax Hygge Candle in
Rosewood + Patchouli

LEAST FAVORITE THINGS
Alligators
Heights

FAVORITE THING TO DO
Hang out with my whole family. I would
not trade that for anything!

of accomplishment. All I've ever wanted was for girls to like me. And now that I finally have what's really important to me in my career, it's the greatest feeling up onstage. I left that girl crying beneath the stage before a Jonas Brothers concert in the dust, as my mama would say.

Eric helped me overcome my anxiety left over from my childhood experiences of being bullied by forcing me to confront my fears while loving me the entire time. Our reality show was another incredible form of therapy for which I'm grateful. Knowing that I'm truly accepted by women has healed me forever.

SINGING FOR MY MERMAIDS

Performing for my fans is one of my favorite parts of my career. When I get out there and see the beautiful faces of my fans singing along, I can truly feel the room and all the girl power. I still pinch myself every time I walk out to a couple thousand girls dressed up like me, chanting my name and ready for a good time.

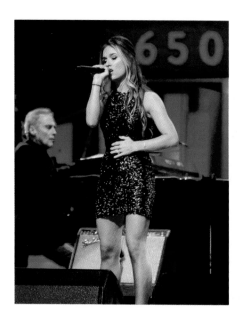

Because I care so much and want to make sure everyone who comes out to see me perform has a good time, I get really nervous right before I go onstage. So I don't like having a lot of people around me. Instead, I listen to a playlist and have a little coffee as I do my makeup. I love this quiet time, as I get really focused and go over the set list in my head.

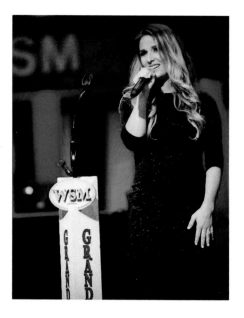

I always have gum in my mouth onstage so that I can keep my throat from going dry, which it tends to do. While performing, I also always have hot tea and lukewarm water on hand. I've literally lost my voice onstage before from drinking ice-cold water. That is a big no-no for singers.

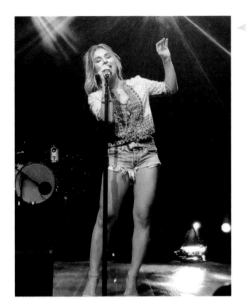

I usually pick out my outfit last minute, but I make sure to always have comfy shoes because I move around a lot. My go-to look is typically cutoffs, a cute top, and booties or high heels. I like to be comfortable. It's all about the hair and makeup anyway.

As soon as I'm ready, I meet up with my band in their dressing room, where we go over the set list together and run through any last-minute tweaks. Then we either have a shot of whiskey or a glass of wine, and— *bam*—it's showtime!

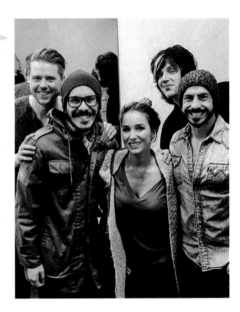

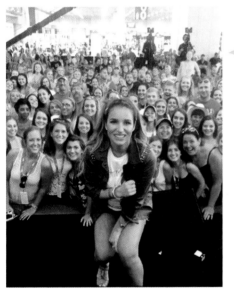

My shows are nontraditional. I do a ton of audience engagement and talk to my fans a lot. I love including everyone as much as possible, because I truly enjoy it and am grateful for everyone's presence.

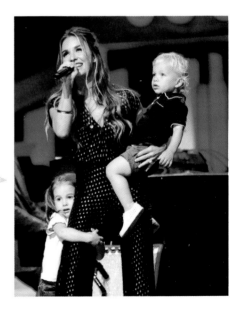

I love having my family with me when I'm performing. They help my confidence, especially my mama. When I'm onstage, I always look over to her for a you're-doing-great smile and nod. I look to my sister for this too—mainly because I know my mama and Sydney will give it to me straight. I would look to Eric, but he always has rose-colored glasses on when it comes to me.

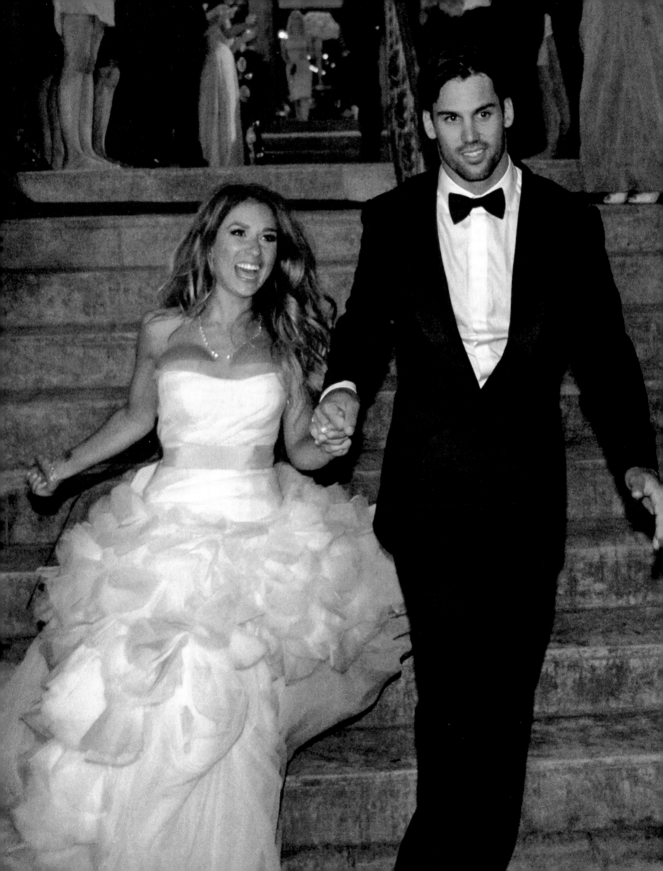

wedding belles

I always thought I would elope somewhere tropical in a sexy mermaid gown with twenty close friends and family in attendance for my wedding. Instead, I ended up saying "I do" wearing a cupcake dress in front of two hundred people in a Catholic church, followed by a reception in a castle!

Oh, and the whole wedding was filmed for an E! special.

No, I was not your typical bride.

As far as weddings go, I was never the little girl who fantasized about getting married. I never dreamed of the big white dress, the flowers, the location, the food. None of that was important to me. I dreamed about my career, what I'd wear onstage while performing for thousands, my band, my music.

Obviously, the right man completely changed my view. Once I met Eric, I didn't give up on my career, but I realized it was no longer the most important part of my life. Still, when

it's a day for you and your man

Make sure and remember your wedding day is about you and your husband-to-be, not about what anyone else wants. Obviously be realistic and don't get upset if not everyone can make it to Thailand if that's where you want to get married. Just keep the focus on you and your man and what makes you the happiest, because this time is yours. Don't let anyone else steal it from you. That can mean anything from appeasing others by doing things you don't feel like doing to letting negative voices take over the narrative. It's *your* day—your thoughts and feelings are the ones that matter.

Eric asked me to marry him, I assumed we'd be engaged for a while. I was in no hurry to get married—not because I didn't love him, but because, well, we were young, and why rush? Eric, though, wanted to be married very quickly.

Suddenly, I was headed for a huge princesslike wedding! Where was the cool musician chick who was going to say her vows barefoot on a beach? I'll tell you where she was—getting fitted for a strapless Vera Wang gown.

The dress, the castle—it felt right with Eric. He was truly my prince, because he had given me my fairy tale. When I got married to him, I wanted to go for it.

LUCKY IN LOVE AND FAMILY

I'm not a planner. I never have been. I'm very quick to make decisions because I just want to get in and out fast. So I always go with my first instinct (and deal with the problems later). I would never make it as a wedding planner. I don't have the patience.

I could *never* have had my big, beautiful wedding without my mom and my sister. They did everything. Now, I know a lot of folks might read this and think, "Ugh!" For a lot of brides, the biggest challenge they face is their families, people who have a very different vision for the wedding and aren't shy about making their wishes clear. I know just how lucky I am that I didn't have a momzilla, sister-zilla, or any other monsters looking to crush the most special event of my life. It was just the opposite: my mom

jessie says
don't be a procrastinator

My mama is probably laughing reading this right now, because I'm the ultimate procrastinator. Once I get around to making a decision, I do it fast. Take my wedding dress: I picked the second one I tried on. I'm all about going with your instincts. But I will say picking a venue wasn't as easy—because I put off dealing with it. We chose ours at the very last minute. If you want a specific venue, caterer, makeup artist, dress, or DJ, you gotta get on it! Once you've decided on an element, lock it in and book it. A year, or however far away your wedding is, might seem like an age, but it comes rolling around fast. Trust me.

and Sydney were angels—with clipboards, lists, Pinterest pages, and cake samples.

Even with my mom and sister doing all the legwork and my don't-overthink-it attitude, there were still moments leading up to the wedding where I felt overwhelmed. It's inevitable when planning a wedding. You haven't used a mailbox in years and suddenly you're sending out a hundred invitations. Or you need to pick flower arrangements. Take deep breaths and try not to get too stressed out. When things get messed up or don't turn out as you thought, which is inevitable, roll with the punches. Stay focused on what really matters to you.

What mattered to me was that our wedding be a true reflection of Eric and me: traditional without being afraid to break some rules. For instance, we spent the night before our wedding together, even though traditionally you're not supposed to. At our rehearsal dinner, Eric said he didn't want to spend the night apart from me, that he wanted to go to sleep together and wake up on our wedding day together. I felt exactly the same way.

So after we woke up and had our coffee in bed, I headed to the venue to get ready for our special day and Eric stayed in our home with his guys to get ready. For the service, my mom gave me a rosary that she wrapped around my bouquet and a handkerchief that belonged to my great-aunts, those little Italian ladies of Independence, Louisiana, who were there that day with me in spirit.

I was so anxious and nervous in the limo headed to the church to marry my prince. But as soon as I got there and Steve took me by my arm, I began to relax a little more. I'm so grateful that he entered our lives, because through him and my mom, I really learned what it means to have a great marriage. I don't think I've ever even seen them have a fight. They're still, to this day, madly in love with each other. He walks through the door from work, and my mom jumps on him. They're so happy.

groom's gift

A really nice watch, engraved with the wedding date or something meaningful, is a traditional groom's gift, which is great if you can afford it—and your groom wears a watch.

For Eric, I did a boudoir shoot and had a book made from the sexy photos that he could keep in his closet to look at when I'm out of town.

If you've broken the bank on your wedding (who hasn't?) and are looking for an affordable option, get two gorgeous, cozy robes embroidered with your new last name and his last name on each robe. Give him his robe in a box with a cutesy framed picture of you wearing your robe, so he knows his is one of a pair. Perhaps add a card that says, "I'll be wearing this as I'm getting ready in the morning to become Mrs. So-and-So." You'll be able to keep those robes in your bathroom forever as a reminder of your incredible wedding day.

Eric is so much like Steve. They're kind and nonjudgmental midwestern men. But I wouldn't have had that example—I wouldn't have known better—if Steve hadn't come into our lives. Even my sister's husband, Anthony, is a nice midwestern guy. It's like we both married men similar to what we had grown up around (thank God). I was so proud to have him, dressed in his air force uniform, escort me to the altar.

When I walked into the church and saw Eric waiting for me at the altar, I really knew how much he loved me, because he was crying and so emotional. I knew I was walking down the aisle to someone who would love me for the rest of our lives. That moment is clear as crystal in a day that otherwise went by so fast.

PARTY TIME

It wouldn't be a normal wedding without a couple of hiccups, and we certainly had ours. But all in all, looking back, it was a beautiful event—and one that, again, reflected who we are as people. Yes, we had a pretty traditional affair in a lot of ways (think my big southern dress), but we also included little elements to make it our own.

Eric and I wanted our wedding to be elegant but also really fun. I like things to be nice and done well while still keeping it real. So, although

jessie says

beauty musts for any bride

* **WEAR FALSE EYELASHES ON YOUR WEDDING DAY.** They make your eyes pop and you don't have to worry about running mascara. Just wear them.

* **MAKE SURE TO GET AN EMERGENCY BRIDAL KIT.** Lots of places make them, and the Knot has a DIY version you can do: pack in a small bag safety pins, tissues, mints, extra bobby pins—all those little things that really do come in handy.

* **DEODORANT AND TAMPONS.** I started my period the day of my wedding, and even though my cycle is as regular as clockwork, my period was not at the top of my mind the morning of the biggest commitment of my life. So I had to go around asking different girls at the wedding if they had any extra tampons. I also was sweating like crazy.

the reception took place in a castle, we had beer pong, which was a blast. When it came to the menu, I insisted on a crawfish boil, passion iced tea, and peach salad—all foods that reflect what I like and who I am, because those are the touches that make a wedding personal.

Don't be afraid to put your unique stamp on every element of your wedding. I'm a southern girl at heart, so I decided at my wedding I wanted people to drink out of mason jars for the down-home feel. At Walmart I bought twenty-four crates of mason jars at fifteen bucks a crate. Then I wrapped twine around each one and attached a name tag, so the glass doubled as a place setting and keepsake from the event. You don't have to spend a lot of money on things like that. The important thing is to make it yours.

WHERE TO SAVE

Don't spend a lot of money on decor items. If you're creative, you can find plenty of knickknacks at large discount stores like Target, Walmart, Pier 1 Imports, or HomeGoods. I found so many cute and different little things at thrift stores to jazz up the space so it felt less like an events venue and more like a party.

WHERE TO SPEND

The food. People *always* remember the food. You don't need to serve lobster tails and filet mignon. We had Cajun-themed food, because my whole family's from Louisiana. You can serve big platters of pasta. It doesn't matter the type of cuisine, only the quality and that there's plenty to go around. There's nothing worse than a party without enough food.

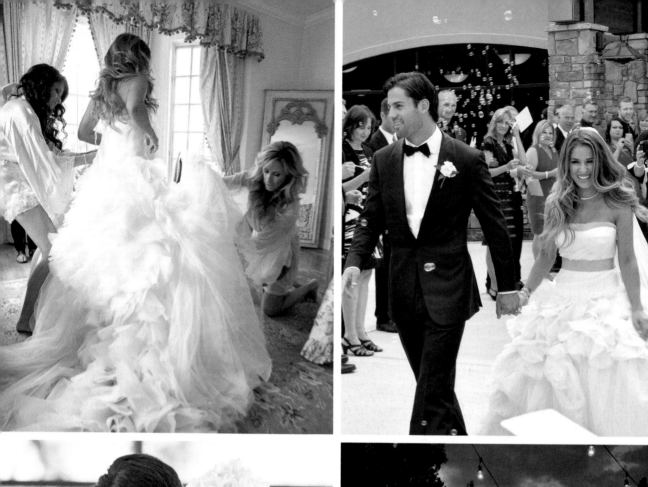
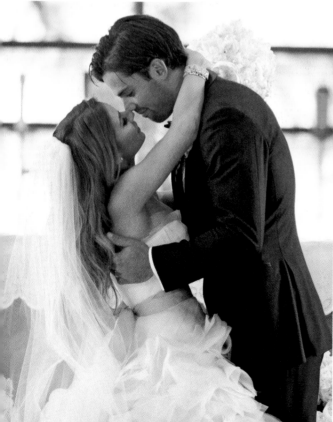
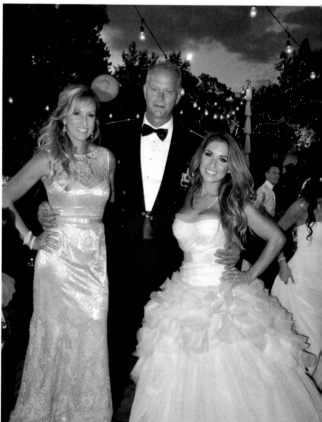

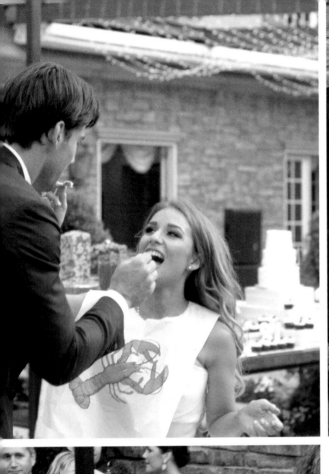
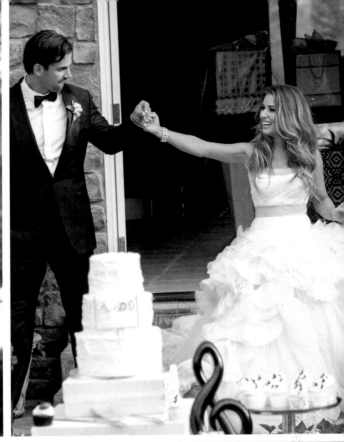
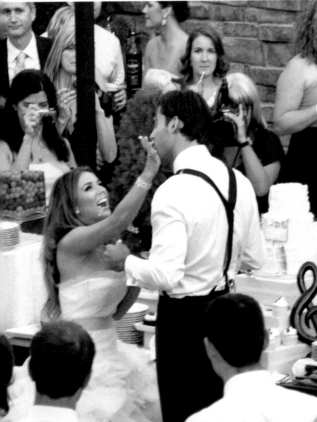
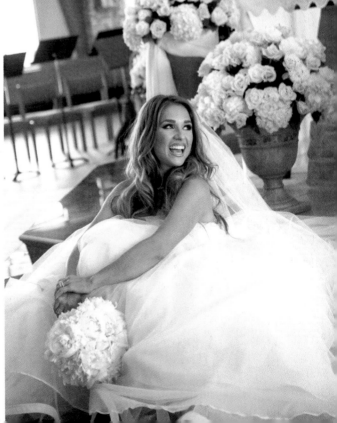

Of course, the other place to splurge is on how you look, from your hair to your shoes, because come on! I've been doing my own hair and makeup forever, because it's part of my career, so I was in a unique position. I colored my own hair for the wedding, and my best friend and makeup artist, Jessica, and I did my hair and makeup together the day of the wedding.

Jessica's done my makeup a million times. Still, I got a little flustered getting ready the morning of the wedding, because I didn't think my makeup was looking right. I was sweating so badly, because when I get nervous, I just sweat. I also got my period that day, which didn't help any. Add to that the cameras filming all around me! But even if you're getting married in a field with twenty of your closest people, your wedding is a really big day. And if you don't have a breakdown at some point, then you ain't normal.

READY, SET, GO! DESTINATION WEDDING THE RIGHT WAY

My sister did her destination wedding right. When Sydney and Anthony got married, they chose sunny Cabo San Lucas—and it was perfection.

The seeds of her destination wedding were planted three years earlier, when Eric, Jessica, Sydney, and a few of our good friends headed down to the popular spot in Mexico for a group vacation. One afternoon, we went to Flora Farms, which is one of the most beautiful restaurants in the world. Every time we're in Cabo, Eric and I go to the farm-to-table eatery, where every ingredient is right from its garden. While the sun began to glow orange through the sunflowers growing all around us, Sydney announced to our table, "I'm getting married here."

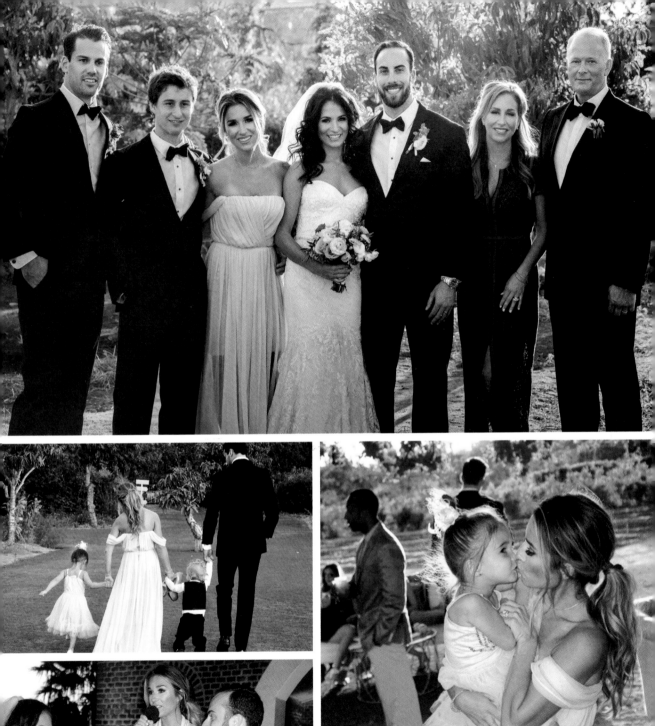
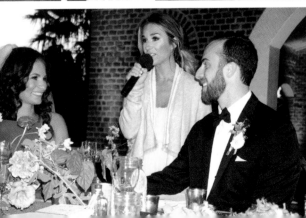
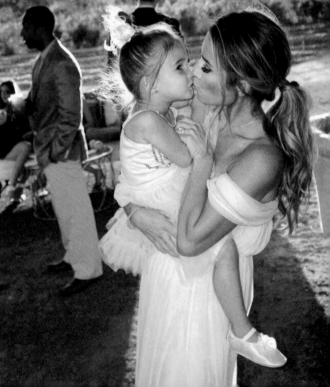

That stuck with her, and when she found the right man, she did just that.

Sydney's wedding was completely different from mine. I actually think hers ran smoother than mine did. Maybe it wasn't as stressful because it wasn't my wedding day, but I also believe that out-of-town weddings can be a lot easier. These venues (at least the good ones) make the whole experience so easy. It starts with the planning. The choices are narrowed down—three options for flowers, a few set menus to choose from, etc.—which eliminates a lot of the stress. If you're already a high-strung person, this is the way to do it. Then once you arrive, they take care of everything. I can't recommend it enough.

jessie says

travel notes

If, while traveling, you go to a restaurant or resort that is beautiful and the food is delicious, ask if it does weddings (even if you're single). File the location away for when you're ready to tie the knot.

Sydney, who was very at peace and happy the entire time we were in Mexico, still found ways to put her own touch on the event. For example, we handed out beach-bag-themed gifts bags with sunscreen and other fun beachy stuff.

Naturally, Jessica and I did Sydney's hair and makeup. Like her wedding, her look was completely opposite of what I had. We have different coloring. Sydney has dark curly hair and big green eyes, which Jessica and I played up. She also wore a fitted mermaid gown that complimented her tiny waist. It's the most beautiful Sydney's ever looked. Another difference: I designed all the bridesmaids' gowns for my wedding, but we got Vivianne's flower girl dress off Amazon! She looked precious.

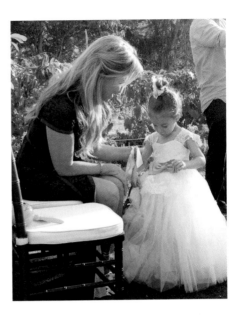

What struck me about Sydney's wedding is that even if you go the destination route, the family element can still be very much present. The majority of our family was able to go to Sydney's wedding, and still to this day my siblings and I talk about how it was some of the most fun times we've ever had all together! Yes, not everyone you invite will be able to go. But that doesn't mean you have to do it in your hometown just so everyone can attend. Remember, it's *your* day. Some people love the opportunity for a vacation. Your friends and family will make it work if they can. And if they can't, you have to be okay with that.

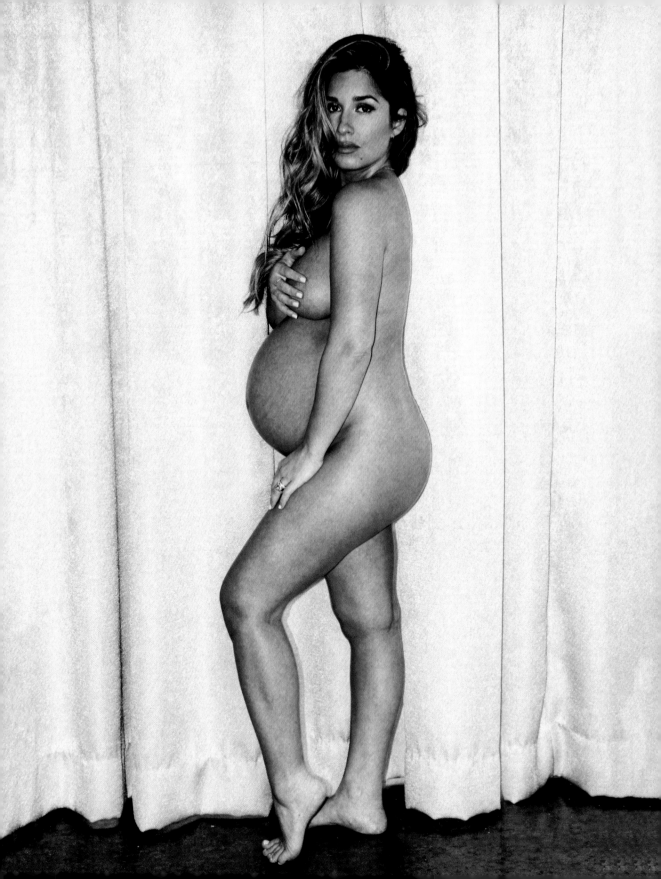

knocked up fast

Eric and I honeymooned in Hawaii, which was pure bliss. In general, Eric and I are not the kind of people who like to do a lot of adventuring when we go on vacation. We don't need to bungee jump off bridges or swim with sharks. No, we stay at the hotel, lounge around, soak up the sun all day, and just eat and eat and eat. That's what we do on vacations: we lie around and look forward to our next meal.

That's exactly what we did in Hawaii. When we came back to Colorado, I guess we brought back those blissed-out honeymoon vibes, because no more than four or five days after our return, we made Vivianne.

We weren't planning on that happening. I wasn't on birth control, but my periods have always been extremely accurate so I knew the exact three days I was ovulating. During one of those days right after our honeymoon, Eric wanted to be together. I asked him if he was sure. I knew my periods were

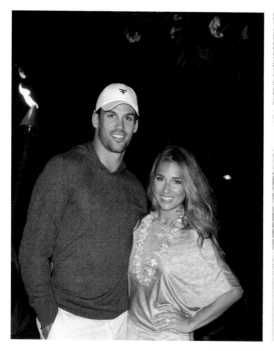
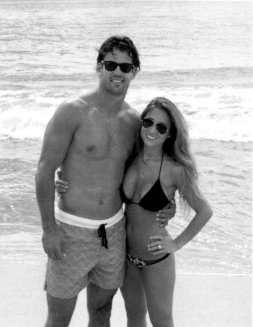

like clockwork, but I had no idea how fertile I was—or he was. "But if you want to play with fire," I said, "these are the days we're playing with fire."

So we played with fire, and a few weeks later, on July 22, exactly one month after our June 22 wedding (and the first day of my last period), I found out I was pregnant.

BUN IN THE OVEN

As soon as I found out I was pregnant, Eric was excited and I was really freaked out. There's a line from the movie *Overboard,* with Goldie Hawn, where her character's mother says to her, "If you have a baby, you won't be the baby anymore." That perfectly summed up how I was feeling: *I am no longer the baby. It's now time to be a grown-up.*

Up until that point I could be as selfish as I wanted. When it was just

Eric and me, I could sleep until noon, lounge around, get my nails done, travel at my leisure, do my own thing. With a baby, that would all go away. It came as a big moment of shock.

No sooner had the shock worn off (a little) than the morning sickness kicked in. I know morning sickness is what they call it, but that name doesn't really do what I experienced justice. I threw up every single day for four and a half months. Sometimes twice a day. The feeling of nausea that sent me running to the toilet all the time was similar to that feeling of when you're so hungry you feel like you're going to puke. The only way to calm my stomach was to fill it up and fill it up fast. I would shove anything I could in my mouth—bread, cinnamon rolls, carbs of any shape or size. Anything to make the nausea stop.

Because of that, I gained 55 pounds with Vivianne. That might not seem like a lot, but I got up to 163 pounds when I had never weighed more than 116 pounds in my entire life. I'm five-foot-one and typically weigh between 110 and 114 pounds. I'm very petite, so that kind of weight put a lot of stress on my body. My boobs got so massive my back was killing me. The shock to my joints was, well, shocking.

Five months into my pregnancy, I developed carpal tunnel and tendonitis. I was hitting nerves in my arms and my hands would go numb. It was so bad I couldn't even put on mascara without my hand shaking and going completely numb. It was so intense I had to wear wrist guards.

On top of being so huge myself, I was carrying a large baby. I was born at nine pounds, five ounces, and Eric was eight pounds, fifteen ounces, so I knew a big baby was in my future. I was so uncomfortable.

Oh, did I mention I also got the H1N1 virus—otherwise known as swine flu—*twice*? It was a hell pregnancy. Vivianne kicked my ass. Out of all three pregnancies, Vivi's was the hardest. Because I felt so sick and had no energy, I did nothing in terms of exercise (another reason I gained all that weight). When I was pregnant with my second, Eric II, whom we call

I just love traditional southern names. In the film *Divine Secrets of the Ya-Ya Sisterhood*, I loved the way the father of Ashley Judd's character, Viviane Joan Abbott Walker, said her name: "Vivi-anne Walker." When we knew we were expecting a girl, I asked Eric what he thought about the name Vivianne. "I love it," he said. With Bubby, Eric always wanted to have a son named after him, which is very traditional and sweet. With Forrest, the movie *Forrest Gump* is my favorite movie of all time. The name is so beautiful and just embodies the South to me.

Bubby, I wasn't sick. I threw up every day for one week—just one week—and that was it. I had only one food aversion with Bubby: pork. I didn't necessarily exercise when I was carrying him, but I walked a lot—and I was running after little Vivianne. Plus, I worked. All of that helped me to burn calories and keep me from gaining the destructive weight I did with my first pregnancy.

I think if you pay attention to your pregnancies, you can learn a lot about the personalities of your children while they're still inside of you. Vivianne's pregnancy was my toughest—and girlfriend still kicks my ass in real life too. My pregnancy with Bubs was easy, and he was an easy, easy baby.

With Vivianne, my little stubborn girl: there would be days I wouldn't feel her move or kick, and it would stress me out to no end. "Come on. Move!" I'd command my belly, consumed with anxiety that something was wrong. I wasn't beyond calling my ob-gyn at eight o'clock at night and insisting I had to come in for an ultrasound, because I was in such a panic. My doctor's nurse, an angel who put up with my craziness, said, "She's perfectly fine. She's just being stubborn." Whereas with Bubby, if all of a sudden I had that thought of "I haven't felt him in forever," that very second he would kick, as if to say, "I'm here, Mom. Don't worry about it."

To this day Bubby is very sensitive to my emotional state. We play a game where if I pretend to cry, he comes up and he puts both his hands on my face and gives me kisses. Vivi's a tough, special girl. She makes me work for her—and I don't mind.

My pregnancy with Forrest was somewhere in the middle. I threw up with him only once but was so nauseated for the first ten weeks that I wished I could have thrown up for some relief. The other hard part with Forrest was how low he was for the last few months; apparently he was getting himself ready for birth early on by sitting low in my pelvis. Because of this, I had to pee pretty much every twenty minutes. Other than that he was a dream pregnancy and took it easy on his mama.

But there was something very different about my pregnancy with Vivianne. The first pregnancy for anyone is tough. It's your first time growing a human being in your body.

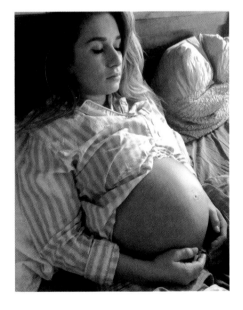

It's exhausting, mentally and physically. You don't know what's going on with you and feel like there's an alien in your body. It's unlike anything you've ever done. With Vivi, though, I felt like we were one. I was very connected to her. So even though it was a pretty crazy pregnancy and a lot went down, I still enjoyed it.

In a weird way, I loved being pregnant with my daughter. Despite all the discomfort and nerves, there was a

I always say: if you have great hair and makeup, then the rest looks put-together. You can be comfortable without looking sloppy. I live in leggings and T-shirts (even when I'm not pregnant). Wear a nice pair of black leggings, a V-neck, and cute little slip-on tennis shoes; roll your hair; put on some aviators and cool earrings; and you'll look and feel great—even if you're at the end of your pregnancy.

blissful side of taking in the fact that I was going to be a mommy. "How lucky am I," I thought, "to be able to grow this person and start our beautiful family?"

NFL WIVES AND NESTING

While I got bigger and bigger with Vivi, I completely cut back with work. Let me rephrase: I did nothing. Because physically I couldn't do anything. It wasn't such a big shift, since my music career had already slowed down a lot after moving to Denver, and we had finished filming our first season of our reality show.

I really nested. Because it was wintertime, the fireplace was always going and so was the oven. I made so many soups, stews, and baked goods. Curling up in front of the fire, I wore lots of Victoria's Secret pink pajamas (button-up ones with the little bow) and lots of big, fuzzy slippers. I hibernated while I waited for my baby to get here.

I decided to take this time to fully embrace being a football wife. In the time Eric and I have been together, he's been on a couple of teams. But there was nothing like the Denver community. The women were fantastic. The events were fabulous. Everything about being a Bronco wife was wonderful. Nothing compares.

Some of the greatest memories I have of being part of the NFL organization come from our time living in Colorado. The events held for the team were like something out of a movie or a fairy tale—or both! The Broncos' owner, Pat Bowlen, and his wife, Annabel, hosted a big Christmas party at their house when the team was in the playoffs and set to go to the Super Bowl. It was the fanciest party at the fanciest house I've ever seen. As pro athletes and their wives, everyone at the event was very well-off. But this was a whole other level. As we walked into the mega-mansion in our Christmas finest, servers greeted us with flutes of champagne. When I have a party, I'm waiting on everybody and making the food. Not here. The sit-down dinner was a delicious and elegant affair where Mrs. Bowlen got up to give a fabulous, welcoming speech.

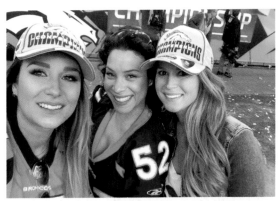

The parties were great, but the other Broncos wives were really what made my time in Colorado special. We all loved one another. It was a true sisterhood. From this group of incredible ladies, I met two of my closest friends. Nikki Colquitt, wife of Broncos punter Britton Colquitt, and Veronica Woodyard, married to Broncos linebacker Wesley Woodyard, are two women I'll be friends with for the rest of my life.

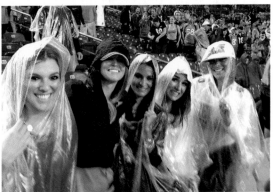

We were all pregnant at the same exact time with our babies. Luckily Nikki already had a baby when I was pregnant with Vivi (she was pregnant with her second). She was really helpful, offering that crucial advice every woman needs from a mom who's already been through the experience. Once while I was over at her house, she was on her knees, folding all the clothes she had just washed for the new baby, when she looked up at me.

"Have you washed all the baby's clothes yet in Dreft?" she asked.

No, I hadn't. I didn't even know that was a thing.

"You have to," she said.

It's such a simple thing, but I would have come home from the hospital to find all the baby's clothes still hanging in the closet with the tags on them.

(Another tip from a mommy friend that I tell all my first-time-mom friends: don't worry about buying a bottle cleaner and sanitizer contraption, which takes up so much space on the counter. It's a waste. Put your bottles in the dishwasher; it does the exact same thing.)

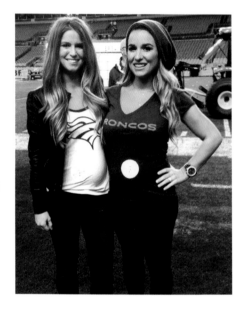

It was really great to have good girlfriends who were contemporaries so I didn't need to be afraid to ask for advice. These women weren't going to laugh at me, think my questions were dumb, or judge that I was going to be a bad mom for not knowing you have to wash your baby's clothes before she wears them.

Plus, we had a blast being pregnant together. We pampered ourselves a lot. There was a spa in Colorado called Belly Up that was geared toward pregnant women. So you didn't have to say, "I can't lie on my back" during a massage, because they already knew. They knew everything. It was heaven.

I refuse to call myself an NFL WAG (Wives and Girlfriends). I just think that's a dumb name. But it is a sorority mainly because we're all on the same schedule, which revolves around—what else?— football.

- ★ Every football wife knows that Tuesdays are the players' day off, so that means Monday nights are date night.

- ★ Saturday nights the men stay at hotels even in their hometown. When away, the men will most likely go in a group to the nearest fancy steak house to fuel up on protein the night before the big game.

- ★ Right after away games the guys hop on a plane and head right back home, sometimes not getting back until three in the morning. Pretty much every football wife will wake up when her husband comes home to greet him, win or loss. Typically the guys don't want their wives traveling because that means they have to fly home to an empty house. They want their women there when they get home to either coddle them after a loss or praise them after a win.

- ★ There's not a lot of sex going on during football season. The men are so tired and they're saving their testosterone for the field. There's definitely no sex the night or even day before a game. That's part of the reason the men stay in a hotel the night before the games: so they can stay focused on all levels.

- ★ All the women get really sad around the end of July and start of August, because the men go away to training camp, and you don't get to see them or have them home for four weeks.

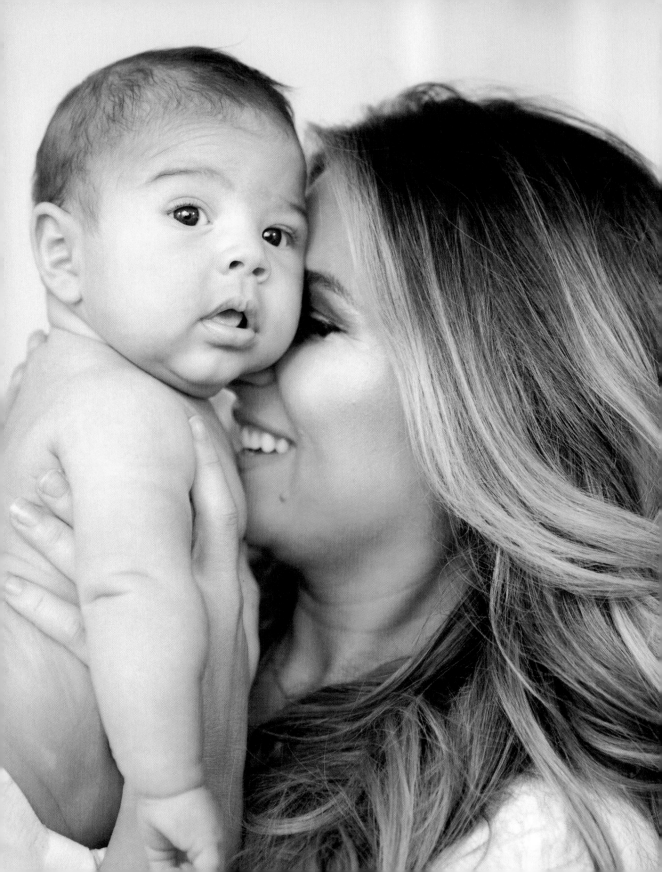

new baby, new mommy

For months leading up to the birth of my first baby, I had fantasies of the delivery process. I watched hundreds of YouTube videos of women pushing out babies and then holding them to their chests in *that* moment. I just knew the moment I held my daughter, Viv, on my chest for the first time would inform the entire future of our loving relationship and bond.

Plus I was sick of being pregnant. After throwing up every day for almost five months, at thirty-four weeks I was put on bed rest and medication because I went into early labor. I got the H1N1 virus and tendonitis and carpal tunnel. Viv kicked me constantly, hitting that vaginal nerve that makes you want to scream. Yes, this little girl kicked my petite five-foot-one ass.

must-have items for your hospital stay

Having gone through labor once before, I was better prepared for the hospital my second time around. Here's what I always tell my girlfriends who are expecting to have ready for when it's go time:

* A long robe and comfy slippers with grips to prevent slipping on slick hospital floors

* Cotton pajamas that button up the front, which are easy to put on and take off

* Massive pads for all that extra fun bleeding after you give birth (most hospitals will provide these)

* Nice big, comfy grandma panties so you don't ruin your fancy ones. You will want to throw these out before you go home.

* A diaper bag for all the baby's items, including a baby onesie, socks, and a hat (most hospitals provide extras as well)

* A mommy bag for all your items

* Your camera

* Your comfy pillow and your husband's comfy pillow and a blanket—hospital couches are not the most relaxing place!

* Toiletries/body wash/razor so you can feel normal again after giving birth.

* A makeup bag so you feel somewhat cute for those after-the-baby-is-born shots in the hospital.

Mercifully, at thirty-eight weeks, I went into labor again; my doctor said it was time for my baby girl to come into the world.

From the get-go, my labor was nothing like those YouTube videos

I'd watched obsessively. First off, my water didn't break on its own, like you always see in the movies. Instead, the doctor had to do it himself with a big plastic tool—right in front of Eric. This was the moment I discovered Eric is *really* bad with the kind of bodily fluids that are usually part of the hospital experience. This six-foot-three, 214-pound wide receiver for the NFL was on the ground. And the real action hadn't even started yet! (Thank goodness Mama was there to take care of us both.)

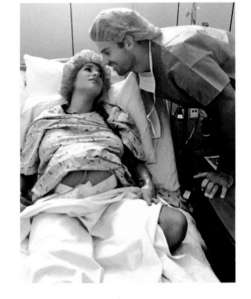

I'll cut to the chase: I spent the next fourteen hours crying from pain and throwing up in between contractions. I'd had an epidural, but I guess it didn't take because I felt *everything*. "I'd have done the hippie thing if I knew this stuff wasn't going to work!" I cried as my mama brushed my hair back and my sister put a cold rag on my forehead, with Eric on the other side, so nervous but still trying to comfort me.

Despite being in more pain than I had ever felt before, my labor never progressed. Viv hadn't moved except to flip over so that she was now face up (I was born this way too). After those fourteen hours of contractions, her head was starting to get stressed. I needed to have an emergency C-section. I was so exhausted I could barely even keep my eyes open. In fact, one of my eyes sealed shut—something I've learned happens to me when I get extremely exhausted. It's a sign my body is starting to shut down. This has happened only twice to me in my life.

Completely terrified, I cried as I watched Eric and Mom put their scrubs on and that blue sheet go up. Eric kept his head by mine, kissing me and saying everything was going to be okay. Little did I know he was

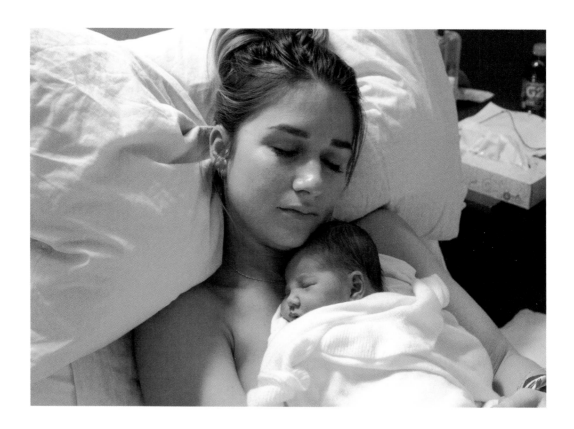

as scared as I was. Before the surgery, he cried in the arms of my mother, who remained a steel magnolia while *her* baby was cut open. That day brought Eric and Mama closer than they already were.

When that baby finally came over the blue sheet, I started to weep—with love for this chunky, beautiful girl and anger because I couldn't touch her. My arms were pinned to my sides because they hadn't yet sewn me up.

"Take these straps off!" I screamed at the anesthesiologist. "Let me hold her!"

But he wouldn't let me.

It seemed like forever before they brought Viv over to me. Funny enough, one of her eyes was sealed shut too from distress. My arms were still strapped down, but I kissed that little face as much as I could, all the while telling her, "I love you. Mommy is here."

NEW BABY BLUES

During the car ride home from the hospital, sitting in the backseat next to Viv in her car seat as Eric drove, I was just so enamored with her. I couldn't believe we had made this little baby together, and now she was coming home with us to start our new lives together. It was a very overwhelming feeling. I cried multiple times a day after Vivi was born. For weeks, which turned into months, I cried and cried and cried. I had a really hard time adjusting to these new feelings. I had never loved anyone as much as I loved this new baby girl. Not even Eric or my mom. She was so fragile and needed so much, and I wasn't sure if I knew how to give her all she needed.

My heightened emotional state mixed with exhaustion and raging hormones was the perfect recipe to develop severe anxiety. I worried even more than I cried. I worried that because we didn't have that first skin-to-chest moment I'd seen on YouTube, our mother-daughter connection was permanently ruined. I was worried someone was going to steal her in the middle of the night. I worried that the red blotches on her skin were signs of a rare medical disorder.

My big mistake was googling everything. When I developed a massive, blistering, and embarrassing cold sore on my lip the day after I came home from the hospital, sure enough, I googled "cold sore" and "newborn" only to find a story about a baby who had died because the newborn's mother had a cold sore and kissed her child! How many times had I already kissed Vivi?!

"I've killed my baby!" I started weeping.

I went so far down the rabbit hole that I forced Eric to take Vivi and me straight back to the hospital. There, the kindly staff talked me off the ledge. They succeeded in assuring me Vivi would live (no small thing), but there was no denying it: I didn't feel like myself.

I'm no doctor, so I don't know if that's clinically what you'd call

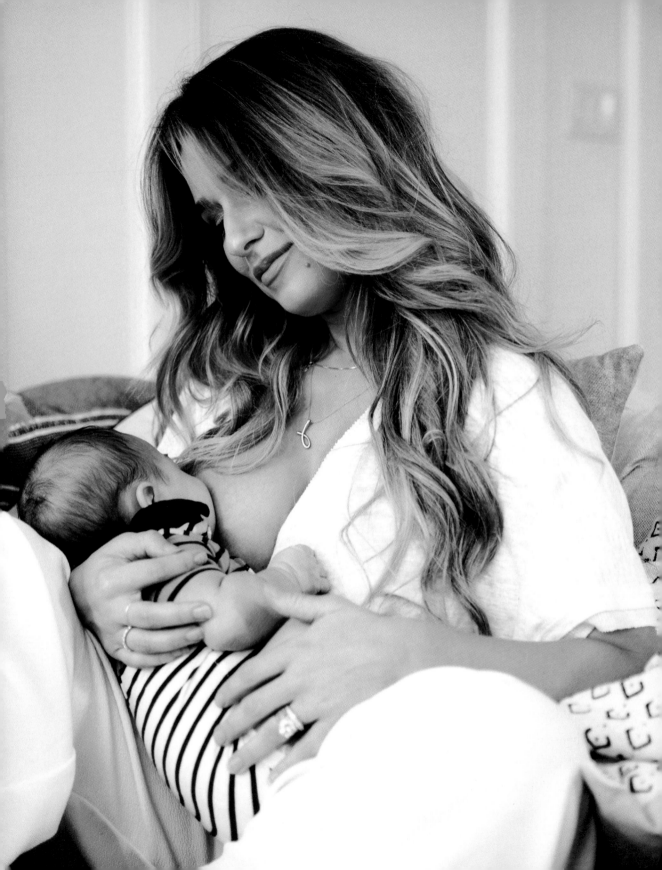

postpartum depression. But there's a lot that happens for new mothers that I think would make anybody have a breakdown. The good thing about my "postpartum" was it didn't interfere with my ability to be a good mama to my baby girl. She was the reason I was able to stay strong and keep going. Whatever stress or pain I was going through disappeared when she was in my arms looking up at me.

Not only was I contending with new motherhood, which is life-changing enough, but a week after Vivi's birth, Eric got a phone call from his agent: he was leaving the Denver Broncos to join the New York Jets.

It was a career high for Eric, who signed a very lucrative five-year contract with the Jets. But for me, it meant immediately packing up my dream home in a city I had loved and lived in for the last four years and finding a new place to live almost two thousand miles away. Let me tell you, in case it's not totally obvious: uprooting your life ten days after having a newborn and when you are still in pain from a C-section is *not* fun.

Thank God Sydney was living with us. I don't know what I would have done without her there. In the very beginning, when Eric was gone at training camp, she would take half the night shift and I would take the other half in my little condo I still had in Nashville. She's such an incredible sister. I know how fortunate I am to have her. When it comes to being a new mom, it's important to take the help that's offered. You can't do it all alone.

THE BLISTERING TRUTH ABOUT BREASTFEEDING

During those early, challenging months of motherhood, the only thing that could make me feel better was being with my daughter. With each passing day, I not only felt so much love for her but also realized I was a natural mother. All of those instincts kicked in, and I knew exactly how to care for my sweet Viv. There was no greater expression of that than when I breastfed her. I just loved nursing Vivi.

Although I *became* a natural at breastfeeding, I didn't start out that way. When I was still in the hospital, the nurses told me that I wasn't producing enough colostrum. The early milk—which has antibodies to protect newborns from disease as well as protein to strengthen them—is usually lower in volume than the milk that comes in later. But apparently mine was *too* low. I felt this huge disappointment come over me. "Great, another fantasy I had about breastfeeding my baby won't be able to happen," I thought.

My anxiety was off the charts and only continued to mount as it looked like I might not be able to produce enough milk at all. Regular milk, which

jessie says
give yourself a break

It isn't easy being a new mom (or any kind of mom, really). But beating yourself up isn't going to make it any easier. No one is perfect. We do the best we can. The important thing to remember is: don't be afraid to ask for help.

Don't feel embarrassed because, I can promise you, every single woman has her own issue as a mother that makes her wonder, "Am I doing this right?" I always say that at the end of the day if you are stressed or feeling guilty, then you're probably on the right track. If you were a bad mom, you wouldn't feel any of that because you wouldn't care enough. (Of course, everything within reason. If you are feeling so anxious or guilty that it is interfering with your normal functions, you should seek help.)

is thinner and usually more plentiful, typically comes in around the third or fourth day of a newborn's life. The last day at the hospital came and went—four days and still no breast milk. I finally decided that we needed to go buy formula just in case this wasn't going to happen. I didn't want my baby to starve.

Then on day five—*bam!*—it was like I was a mama cow. Suddenly I was filling up eight ounces from each boob. There was just tons and tons of milk, so much that we had to buy a separate freezer to fit it all (you can't let that liquid gold go to waste). Not only was the quantity of my milk intense, so was its flow. The force was so strong it would squirt out across the room. "In the olden days, you would have been the village wet nurse for women who couldn't make milk," my mom joked.

I was thrilled for my boobs to be a fountain of milk, but don't get me wrong: breastfeeding still hurt like crazy. I developed mastitis, an infection in the breast that causes massive knots that are just miserable and can cause fevers, and it goes away only by the baby sucking it out or a warm bath. My nipples were blistered, cracked, and bleeding. I remember cringing in pain any time Viv latched on after those first couple of weeks.

But I fought through it and my nipples got tough. Feeding my babies is where I found that mommy bliss. Lying on my side (because my boobs were so big it hurt to sit up), I would stare into their little eyes, pet their heads, talk to and kiss them while they fed and cooed from happy bellies. Those are some of my favorite memories.

That's why when one of my friends told me she was considering giving up on nursing after two weeks, I encouraged her to reconsider. Well, maybe I did a *little* more than encourage. The problem with my friend wasn't her milk supply but rather that the initial pain was making her miserable.

"Get over it," I said. "Get over the blistering. Get over the bleeding. You suck it up, and you feed your baby. You have been given the gift of making milk, so just do it."

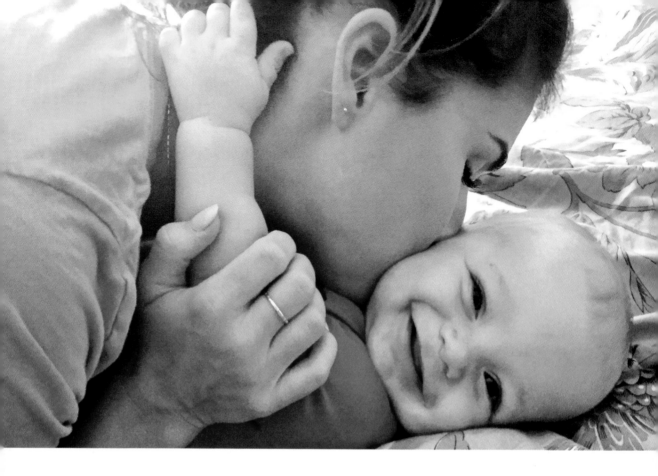

That might sound harsh, but it comes out of love. I wanted my friend—as I want for all mothers—to move past the pain to get to the pleasure. I and countless other women are proof that your nipples toughen up and nursing becomes a truly deep moment of connection. Once I got in the groove, it totally eclipsed that skin-on-skin moment I'd worried so much about missing.

Despite my tough-love stance on breastfeeding for women who *can* make milk, I take the completely opposite stance when it comes to those who *can't*. If your body is just not making milk or not making enough, that's okay. It's the twenty-first century. There is fabulous formula available that can give your baby great nutrients, and there's absolutely nothing wrong with that. In fact, it's the right thing to do.

LET'S HEAR IT FOR THOSE AMAZING DADS

I said I knew Eric would be a great father when I saw him consoling Jenny, our miniature golden retriever, when she was sick. "Damn," I thought at the time. "I picked a good one."

And I did. Never in my life have I witnessed a better dad than this man. He is incredible and inspires me to be a better parent. He will get up in the middle of the night with our children, change diapers, wash bottles, play dolls, read books every night before they go to bed, and take them to work while he gets treatment. None of it is for show or credit. He wants to do these things, because he's naturally a very nurturing person and loves doing it.

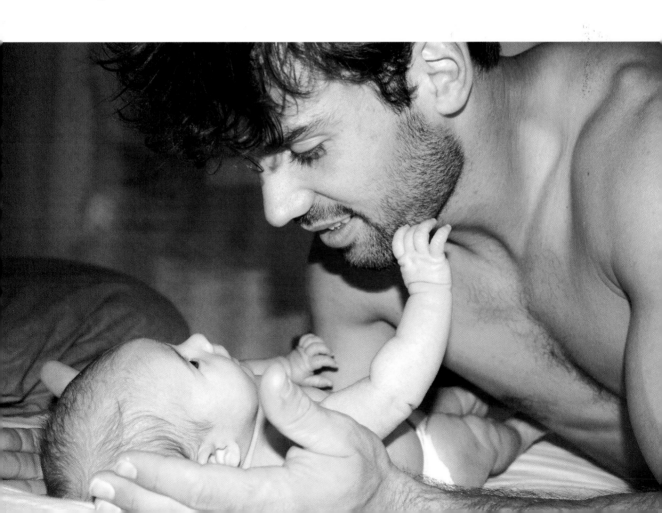

If your partner isn't inherently a caretaker, you can invite him into the experience by taking turns! Get into a routine where when you change a diaper, you say, "The next one's yours, babe." Or "I pumped this milk. How about you do the next feeding?" As mothers, sometimes our default mode is to do everything. Including men in activities that have traditionally been the woman's role allows them the opportunity to bond with their children.

If your man shows resistance or a complete lack of interest, then I would just divorce him and find a new baby daddy. Kidding. Sort of. But honestly, I would not let a man get away with *not* being involved or helping fifty-fifty. This is a teamwork situation. It takes two to make a baby, and it should take two to help raise it.

SECOND-KID STORY

About seven months after Vivi was born, I started to see glimmers of my old self. I was in the groove of taking care of my daughter and had lost a lot of the weight I gained with her. But I never took it completely off, because a month later I got pregnant again with my son.

It terms of my second pregnancy, he took it easier on me than his sister. I threw up for only one week and gained only twenty-eight pounds. I was also much calmer, because I knew what to expect. I knew my body would try to go into early labor again, and I knew I would have a C-section. Sure enough, at thirty-eight weeks, the heavy, consistent contractions began.

Mama and Eric were by my side again. And again, Eric freaked out at the sight of blood. It took three nurses to get him up off the ground after the doctor made the first incision. When my husband came to, there was our son Eric Decker II, all nine pounds of him.

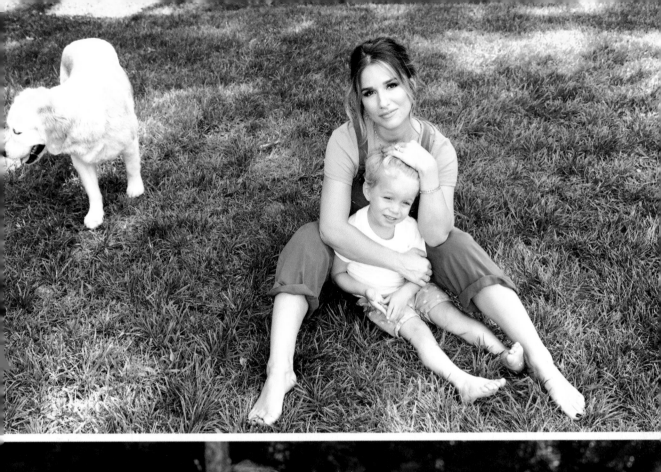
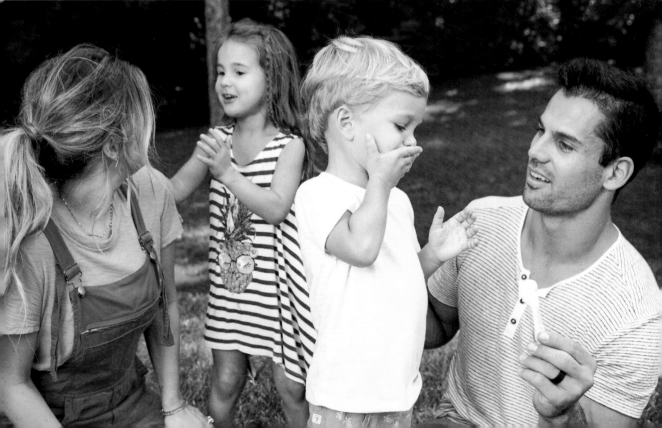

what to bring on the plane when you've got babies

I loved the doctor who delivered Vivianne so much that we flew back to Castle Rock, Colorado, for the births of Eric II and Forrest. Traveling with children is one of the hardest things to do as a parent! Now that I have three children I have learned what to bring to survive.

* Antibacterial wipes to disinfect the dirtiest part of the plane: the tray tables!

* Hand sanitizer

* Baby wipes

* Diapers

* Sippy cups with tops

* Ziplocs with a change of clothes for accidents and to put the dirty clothes in

* Crayons and coloring books

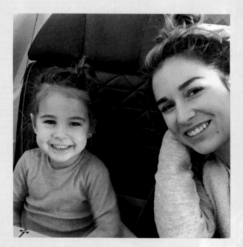

* Blankies and lovies. But whatever you do, *don't lose them* on the plane. They're more important than the passports!

* Snacks (e.g., Goldfish, organic cheese puffs, applesauce squeezers, graham crackers)

* Charged iPads (yes, just do it)

* A handful of emergency suckers. I keep organic dye-free lollipops as a last-ditch effort to calm my kids down. It is called survival! When they just won't behave and are disrupting the entire plane, that's when it's time to whip these suckers out and let them know that if they behave, they will get one.

"Wowwwwww!" everyone in the room said before they began placing bets on his weight.

He was huge, but he had "wimpy white boy syndrome"—yes, that's actually what some people call it when a white male newborn delivered by C-section aspirates on fluid at birth and needs help breathing. The hospital staff rushed off with my son, who was struggling to breathe, so again I didn't get my skin-on-skin moment. This time, however, I was grateful. He needed assistance immediately.

I was taken to my room and told to stay in bed to recover from the surgery I'd just had; they would let me know periodically how my son was doing and eventually take me to see him. Well, it took me only an hour in the recovery room before *my* steel magnolia kicked in. I got out of bed and started to walk, all hunched over from my surgery, across the floor to the NICU. No matter how slow I was moving, I was going to see my baby!

"Mrs. Decker, please!" said a nurse, who tried to guide me back to my room.

"I'm going to see my baby!"

I found my sweet boy all hooked up to wires and oxygen tubes in a plastic box, his chest moving up and down.

"Mommy is here now," I said, holding his little finger.

It was so scary and made my heart hurt for those women whose babies have much more serious issues, like my sister, who had her baby at twenty-eight weeks. I was blessed that my son fought through. We were in the NICU for only a few days until he got his strength to breathe on his own, and we were finally ready to introduce Viv to the newest member of our family.

"Viv, meet baby brother," I said to her.

"Bubby," she responded.

And that was that; this boy will be called Bubby for the rest of his life!

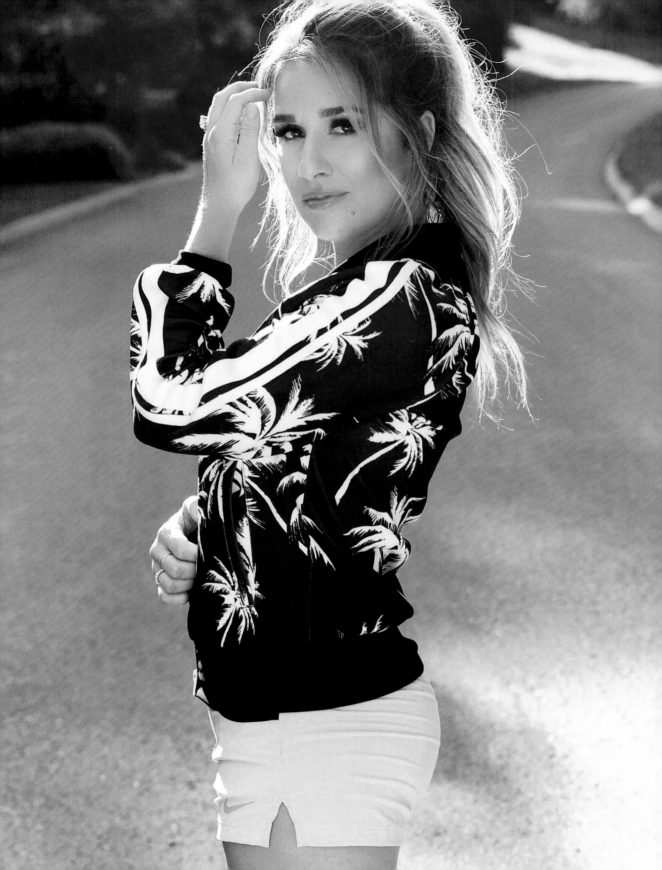

get fit, stay fit

After I had Vivi, I was so focused on being a new mommy and all the new challenges and adventures that it brought that I was too distracted for the first few months to realize just how much weight I had really gained during my pregnancy. As I described in chapter 8, during my pregnancy with Vivi I hit a high of 163 pounds, which was a lot for my five-foot-one frame. Between the water weight and the baby, by the time I left the hospital, I was already down to 145 pounds. But I started out at 116 pounds, so I didn't feel or look like the girl I was used to seeing in the mirror.

None of my clothes fit me, my boobs had grown to size G (which only made me feel bigger), and I didn't plan on hitting the gym any time soon. All of that is pretty normal for a new mom, but of course I only know this now.

Eric, on the other hand, was coming off one of the best

seasons of his career and had gone to the Super Bowl. His face was on a giant billboard in Times Square. I couldn't have been prouder or happier for him, but I also felt the most insecure I had ever felt, sitting at home thirty pounds overweight, nursing, eating, and not sleeping. I was so insecure that I wouldn't go with him to enjoy the New York City festivities.

Perhaps the lowest moment, though, was when we had just moved to New Jersey. I was in a new city with a nursing infant in a temporary housing condo, and Eric was in the city doing a photo shoot for Buffalo Jeans. For its new ad campaign, the denim line chose him and a very sexy Victoria's Secret–type supermodel. Because that's exactly what you need when you have a three-month-old and are thirty pounds overweight: to have your husband spending the day with a girl like that. When I watched the video of the shoot on the internet, I couldn't

jessie says
hold on to that fat . . . for a while

In general, my advice is try not to lose weight—or at least don't do anything extreme—until you are done breastfeeding. I don't say that because of the conventional wisdom that nursing helps lose weight. In fact, I don't think that's even true. At least it wasn't for me. My body held on to extra fat while I was nursing, kind of like a cow. I just think your body is still in recovery and out of whack from the hormones, and there's no reason to mess with it. You have plenty of time to lose weight after you wean your baby.

stop sobbing. The model was lying in his lap with no shirt on! She had a jacket over her, but you could still see her perfect boobs. They were *all* over each other. I knew it was just for the camera and the campaign, but I felt so low and unattractive.

Despite my insecurities, I didn't work out after Vivi was born. That's because I wasn't someone who had ever really worked out. I didn't really know how to diet or what to do in a gym. Pre-pregnancy, Eric called me "juicy" because I was petite but curvy and more on the soft side. Over the course of six months after I gave birth to Vivi, a lot of the weight just kind of dropped off by itself. By the time I got pregnant with Bubby, I was down to 125 pounds.

That's exactly the weight I naturally ended up at seven months after giving birth to Bubby. Up until that point, I didn't diet at all because I wanted to make good milk for him. I stopped breastfeeding Bubby after eight months, but the real reason behind my decision to get serious about fitness was some pictures my mom took of me in a bikini on my birthday. I did *not* like what I saw. That was it!

"Okay, I'm done here," I said. "I'm ready to get back to myself."

GETTING IN SHAPE—
AND STAYING THAT WAY

By the time Bubby turned one, I was down to 110 pounds. That was less than I weighed before the babies, but I wasn't just skinnier. To lose the weight initially, I had to really step up my workouts and diet. In terms of exercise, my brother, John, was the one who really pushed me to start working out. More than just telling me what to do, he *showed* me what to do. His knowledge of fitness and health (as well as his honesty that

I needed to get my butt to the gym) really helped it click for me. He took me to the gym and introduced me to the wonderful world of circuit training that has changed my body and my life.

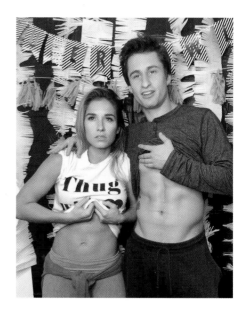

In terms of my diet, I went hard core and restricted myself to 1,000 calories a day. And not just any calories. These were heavy on protein and low on carbs. In addition, I cut out *all* junk. Absolutely no treats! This was just to lose the baby weight I gained. I know for myself, personally, I have to shock my body into losing the weight. When I'm maintaining, it's a whole different story.

The result of all this hard work was that I never felt better. Healthier and more muscular, I decided to make my new eating habits and workouts an ongoing routine (although modified after I was no longer trying to lose weight). Now I'm in the best shape of my life! My body is fitter than it was when I was twenty because I take really good care of it. Here's the regimen that works for me. Tailor it to your own fitness level and always consult a doctor if you are starting to work out for the first time or have serious health conditions.

FITNESS

I've done just about every type of exercise under the sun. I've tried yoga. I've tried Pilates. If you can name it, I've tried it. But once I was introduced to the world of bodybuilding and circuit training, that was it. I found the exercise that works for me. I enjoy the speed of circuit training and the

a picture is worth a thousand resolutions

Take your own before and after pics. Before I started working out, I took pictures of myself in a sports bra and undies and would do side by sides weekly to watch my progress, and I continued to take pictures every week until I hit my goal.

strength of power lifting. (I love heavy weights.)

I started out by watching different videos of circuit-training routines on YouTube. I was looking to see whose bodies I liked, the exercises they did, and how easy it was for me to follow their prompts.

I did get a trainer for a little bit in New Jersey while Eric was playing for the Jets, and I really loved it. I worked with him for only four weeks, but he corrected a lot of things I was doing wrong from my self-taught exercising. For example, I couldn't figure out why my butt wasn't getting more muscular despite a lot of work I was doing on it. It turned out my posture was out of whack, so I was working my quads instead of my glutes. A quick fix and boy were my butt muscles burning!

Hiring a personal trainer for a targeted amount of time to shore up your skills is a great investment. It really does help. While I was getting in shape, I felt like I was working so hard, but some of what I was doing wasn't effective because I wasn't doing it right. I was straining the wrong parts of my body. I also recommend scheduling a couple of sessions, or "tune-ups," with a trainer you like every year, to make sure you haven't slipped back into bad habits or to get new exercise inspiration.

If a personal trainer is not in the budget, find a friend or relative who's passionate about fitness and ask to tag along to the gym with them. Most fitness enthusiasts are more than happy to share their knowledge with anyone who wants to be in better shape.

Part of what attracted me to circuit training is that once I became a mom, I had *no time* to exercise. Heck, a lot of women, moms or not, don't feel like they have any time to work out. Our lives are so busy these days, whether you're a student, a working professional, or a stay-at-home mom. I don't want to be at the gym for ninety minutes. I want to get in and get out. I truly think all you need is thirty minutes of exercise, but it needs to be high impact.

I do thirty minutes of circuit training a day. That's it! When I was first looking to shed my extra pregnancy weight, I added a thirty-minute walk at a fast pace around my neighborhood. If you are new to exercise, walking is a great way to get started. That's how my mom starts her day every morning, and she looks amazing.

I work out at home and at the gym. They both have their benefits. The gym gives you a community and a break from home, which is especially important for new moms, who can feel really isolated. I love the chain Life Time Fitness, which is very mom-friendly. It not only has all the normal amenities of a top fitness club, such as group classes, a swimming pool, and a spa, but it also has a day care for kids. On top of that, each club has a chef who makes fresh diet-friendly dishes and shakes. Every gal deserves to belong to a place like this.

The most obvious benefit of home workouts is the ease. Sometimes there's just not time to get in the car, go to the gym, and do the whole production. And don't believe anyone (like someone on an infomercial) who says you need a ton of equipment. All you need—if you follow my circuit-training workout—is a set of eight- and ten-pound dumbbells. Exercising at home is awesome, because you can do it when your kid's napping.

If you are new to circuit training, start off slowly. Do half of each exercise and work your way up, or start off with a BodyPump class at your local YMCA. I do them all the time and love them.

* 50 jumping jacks
* 20 mountain climbers
* 30 seconds of running with eight-pound dumbbells
* 10 jumping squats
* 15 dead-lifts with ten-pound dumbbells
* 10 donkey kicks
* 20 push-ups

Repeat the entire circuit three times in a row.

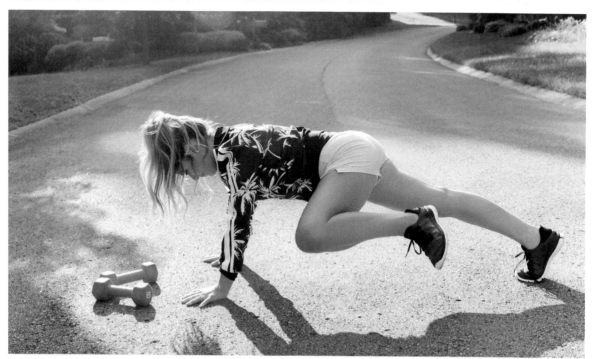

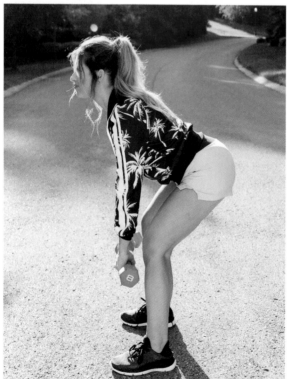

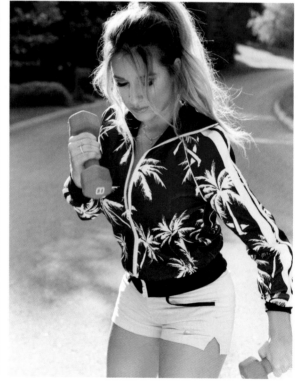

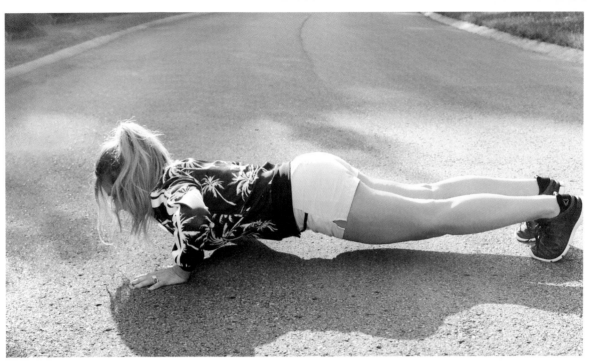

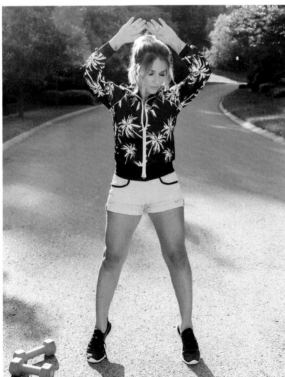

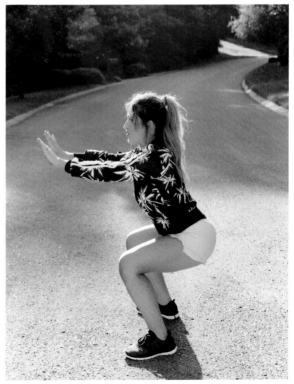

HYDRATION

You know it's always important to drink water, but never is it more crucial to stay hydrated than when you are trying to get back in shape. You need extra water since your muscles are working extra hard. I drink water all day long, but it's always a challenge. The only way I stay on top of it is by drinking out of oversized mason jars with a lid and straw.

My mom orders them for me constantly. I have at least four. I fill them up, add a few slices of lemon, and drink up. That's how I know I'll stay hydrated.

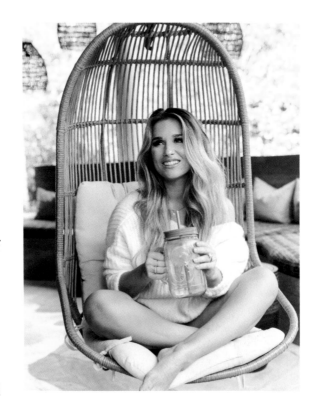

DIET

After I finished breastfeeding my babies, that's when I decided it was time to go hard with a diet. I ate only 1,000 calories a day to drop the extra weight. But I wasn't starving myself. I was drinking protein shakes and eating lean meats and vegetables.

Protein is crucial to keeping up your stamina and building strength while you lose weight. A lot of people skimp on it, and that's a mistake. I drink protein shakes after I work out every single time and aim to have 60 to 75 grams of protein a day.

Now that I'm trying not to lose weight but to instead maintain my target weight, I consume a total of 1,500 calories a day and am definitely not as strict. But I pick my indulgences wisely.

Here's what I eat in a typical day:

BREAKFAST

I'm not a big breakfast person. I don't really believe all the crap about the importance of eating a big old breakfast first thing in the morning. I'm not saying there's a study to prove it (although there probably is since when it comes to dieting there seems to be a study proving everything and the opposite of everything). I'm just letting you know this is how I got and stay thin:

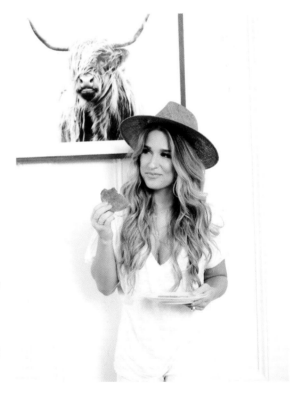

* I have a couple cups of coffee in the morning and then I usually fast until I work out.
* If I do have breakfast, I will have a slice of sourdough toast with organic, grass-fed salted butter. There is nothing wrong with carbs. Your body needs them, particularly if you are working out regularly.
* Immediately after my workout, I have a protein shake with an additional scoop of powdered veggies (just to make sure I get in all my veggies).

LUNCH

Lunch should be your biggest meal of the day. For me, it usually comes pretty quickly after my post-workout shake. Again, I go for a lot of protein. Grilled chicken with riced cauliflower is often on the menu, sometimes with broccoli or maybe peppers and onions. Another fave is marinated flank steak over salad greens.

AFTERNOON SNACK LIST

* Beef jerky stick
* Low-calorie protein bar
* Cheese with honey

DINNER

When you're trying to lose weight, you definitely want to keep it very low carb at night and go heavy on the veggies and protein. I also think it's important not to eat after 6 P.M. When Eric and I are on a diet, we eat at 5:30 P.M.! Chicken Fit-chiladas (page 180) are perfect, because your family will love them. The best thing about these big boys, apart from the taste, is that they're only 150 calories each!

I just can't skip dessert, and there are sneaky ways to get it in even if you are on a strict diet. A handful of strawberries sometimes works to satisfy that sweet tooth, but I also love Smartcakes, which are only 38 calories each with no sugar and 4 grams of protein!

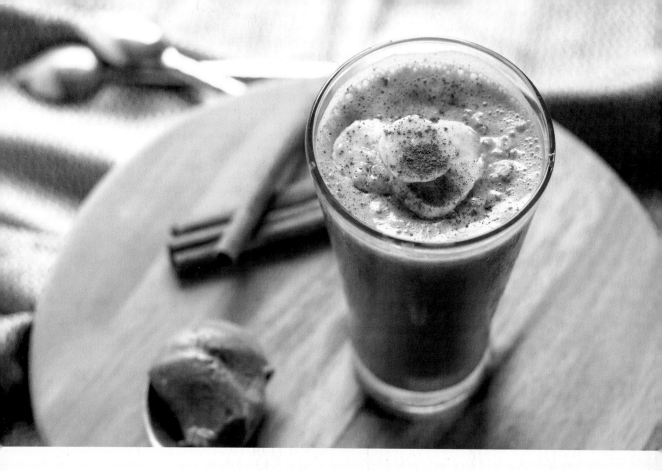

jessie's homemade shake

MAKES 1 SHAKE

Eric initially turned me on to this protein shake, but I altered the recipe to suit me, because he's a big guy and a pro athlete—he needs a lot more calories than I do.

2 cups almond milk

1 heaping tablespoon almond butter

1 dash cinnamon

½ banana

1 serving low-calorie, low-sugar, organic chocolate protein powder (it should contain at least 18 grams of protein per serving)

1 cup ice (or as much as you like)

Add all the ingredients to the jar of a standing blender. Blend and enjoy!

NOTE: If you are breastfeeding, add ½ cup of dry oats, which is great for stimulating milk production.

TREATS

I've never been a big drinker. My body doesn't love alcohol. So that's definitely not where I want to spend my calories. Cookies, on the other hand . . . I have a cookie *every* day, and I will never cut that out. But I don't indulge with some piece-of-crap cookie. No, it's got to be good. I also like to go as natural as possible, because it's harder to process artificial ingredients (especially if you've been cutting them out). Whenever I eat stuff that's full of crap ingredients, I immediately get bloated. So have the sweets without sending your gut into protest. For one of my go-to cookie recipes, try my Chocolate Chip Cookies (page 185).

SCALE ON

I weigh myself *every* morning. I know, I know. Current wisdom states you *shouldn't* do that. But I think it's good to know where you're at with your body. Obviously there are times I ignore the scale, like when I get my period or if I travel (I hold on to water and swell a lot from air travel). In general, though, I want to know if I've gained weight. All of us have certain times of the year that are diet busters. For a lot of folks it's Christmas. For me it's late March through the beginning of May, because it's Eric's birthday, Vivi's birthday, Forrest's birthday, my birthday, my sister's birthday, and, last but not least, my mom's birthday. That's a lot of celebrating—and a lot of cake. When I see the numbers on the scale creep up, I know it's time to start cutting back on the cookies and hitting the gym that much harder. So don't hide your scale and pull it out only when you're already at that number where it'll be so hard to get back to one you're happy with. Be a health rule breaker like me and take control!

KIDS AND EATING

Keeping my kids fed and happy (without losing my mind) is all about having a well-stocked pantry and a bunch of go-to meals. When you have a family, making sure you always have extras of your staples around is vital. Who hasn't run out of peanut butter, or the yogurt has expired, and you've got to make the kids' lunch for tomorrow morning? That's why I always keep a loaf of bread and ground meat in the freezer. And lots of cans of beans—all kinds of beans, from green beans to baked beans to white beans—because you can make so many different things with them.

When I don't have time to go grocery shopping and the kids are hungry, it's stressful and I need something simple, fast, and tasty. That's often chili. I have probably six or seven different versions. There's turkey chili, bison chili, beef chili, and seven-can chili. I learned the last one from a girlfriend of mine. All you do is sauté ground meat with salt, pepper, and chili powder. Then you dump in seven cans (corn, green beans, tomato soup, Ro-Tel, and three cans of beans), let the whole thing simmer for a

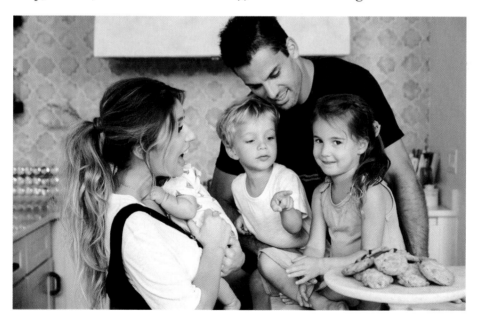

little bit, and it's done. That's it! In fifteen minutes flat, you can have a meal that everyone will devour. And you get all your vegetables. It's perfect.

Another one of my last-minute emergency meals is naan pizza. You can find this round Indian bread in the frozen section of Whole Foods and Trader Joe's. It is another freezer staple in my house. I brush each round with a little olive oil, smother with mozzarella cheese, add whatever my kids like (pepperoni, mushrooms, tomato slices), toss it in the oven for five minutes—and again, that's it. Dinner's on the table.

NOTE: *It's impossible to make homemade meals all day long for your kids. You can think you will, but trust me, you won't. I'm not advocating microwaving those bright orange packages of macaroni and cheese, but you can find prepared foods that are healthy to supplement the meals you do make. I give Bubby kale bites and organic chicken nuggets, which he loves and I can feel good about him eating.*

LEARNING TO BE HEALTHY

Growing up, I was never allowed to drink soda. We also never had colorful cereals. I figured it was because my parents were no fun.

My mom didn't want us consuming soda or certain breakfast cereals because they were full of sugar. When we did have treats, they were like pretty much everything else my mom served us—made from scratch at home. That way she always knew what we were putting in our bodies, which as an adult I understand was one of the greatest things she did for us. Now there's a lot of discussion around the dangers of processed food, but not when I was a kid. Mama was ahead of her time.

Now don't get me wrong. I'm not a crazy health nut. But I have educated myself as much as I possibly can, especially when it comes to what I'm putting in my children's bodies. My children are not allowed to have soda—and they won't as long as they're living under my roof (unless it's a little organic ginger ale for a tummy ache when they're old enough). When I serve them apple juice or grape juice in the morning, I cut it with an equal amount of water.

I'm not totally psycho about all of this stuff. I don't let my kids have anything with added sugar at home, but I will take them to McDonald's for a Happy Meal because kids need to be kids! But most days begin with Eric cutting up fresh fruits and berries for the children's breakfast that also includes organic whole wheat toast with grass-fed butter and scrambled eggs. Then the rest of their meals are similarly healthy.

The only thing I am totally anti is color dye in my kids' food. This is something I had absolutely no clue about until Vivianne started having major allergic reactions to certain foods. I took her in to the allergist, who told me to give her Benadryl when she had a reaction. Within the same conversation, however, he also told me to try and get the dye-free Benadryl in case she has an adverse reaction to the red coloring. I sat there baffled and had no idea what the doctor meant, so I went home and did my research and was scared by what I found! There were claims of connections to behavioral issues and cancer. And what I didn't realize was how many foods contain these dyes. They are in everything from breakfast fruit bars to children's toothpaste— all things that are supposed to be good for

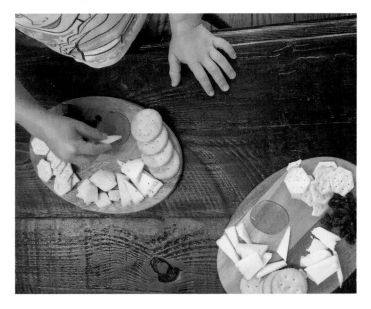

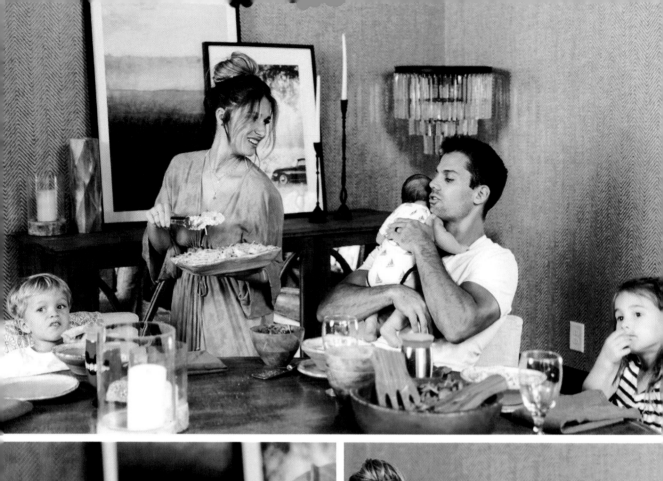

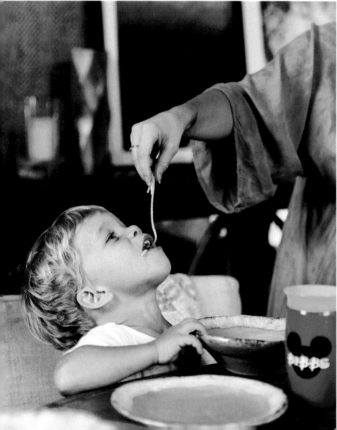

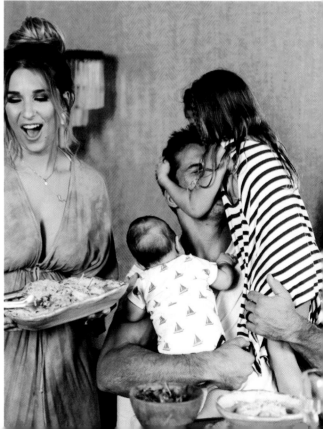

your kids! That's why now I read the ingredients like a hawk and take a pass whenever I find artificial dyes on the list.

MAKE MEALTIME FUN TIME

I went to the house of a friend, and she was giving her three-year-old son lunch. She served him a peanut butter sandwich at the dining room table on a big white china plate. Not a kid's plate, and there was no kid's cup. Nothing fun.

I asked the little boy, "Where's your kid table?"

He looked at me, confused. "I don't have one," he answered.

I decided at that moment I would give him one for Christmas.

It's the little things that make mealtime fun for kids. Get your kids brightly colored plates and trays, forks and spoons, and sippy cups with straws that have their favorite characters on them. Bubby loves to plop down at his plastic Mickey Mouse table and chair to snack. I don't care if it doesn't look pretty. You're only a kid once.

I don't think it's a big deal to let your kids watch cartoons while they eat. I know a lot of people are opposed to television during mealtime. In some cases, it can become a source of overeating. But in my family, it helps me get my kids *to* eat. A little distraction helps Bubby and Viv to finish their breakfast.

That works for us, and I put on their cartoons for breakfast and lunch. But at dinnertime, we don't do that. Dinnertime is family time. Almost every single night, I make a home-cooked meal, and we sit around the big table together. We say our prayers, enjoy the food, and talk to one another. The kids look forward to it. They like to talk about their day just as much as we do.

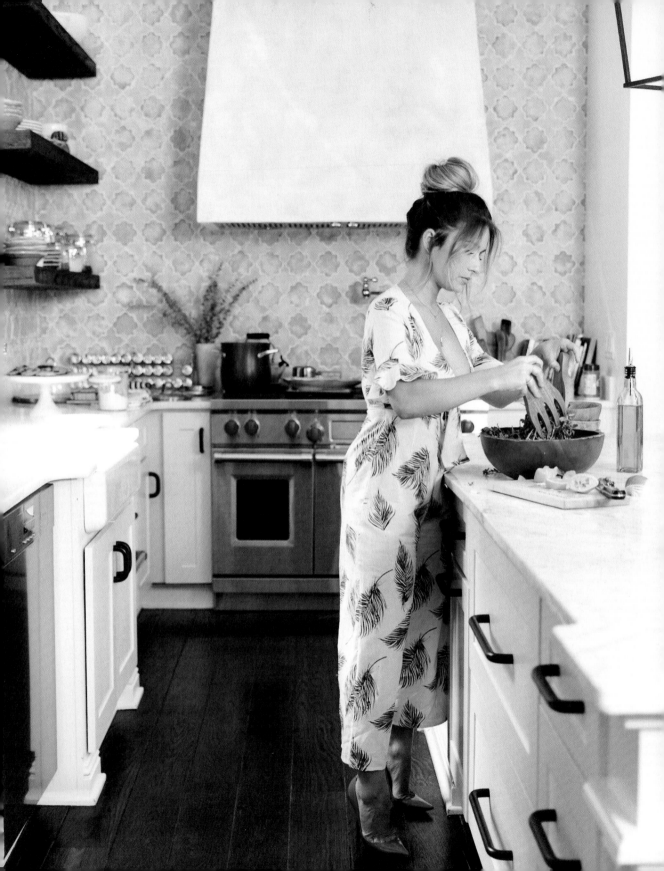

homemakin' and presentation

I was taught by my mother that the secret to making something nice—whether it's your home, a party, or a pastry—is presentation. She always gave me the example of a "presentation" she learned in a college class. Her professor grabbed a piece of cake, threw it down on his desk, and asked, "Do you want to eat this cake?" Everyone in the room shook their heads no. Who would want to eat a piece of cake smashed flat on a desk? Then he brought out another identical piece—this one on a beautiful platter all put together nicely—and asked the same question. The answer was obvious.

I was raised by this rule and still live by it. Sometimes

when I make Eric and myself afternoon lattes, I will put them in beautiful, fancy white cups with saucers underneath. When I have guests over, even good friends whom I see all the time, I light all my candles (including the one in the guest bathroom). It doesn't have to be elaborate, time-consuming, or expensive to bring something special to the moment. When people stay at our home, I think it's nice to put bottled water by their bed and other small useful items, like an eye mask and slippers. I always have samples from my clothing or beauty line that I leave on the bed for when my girlfriends arrive. It adds a nice touch to make folks feel welcome.

But you don't need your own fashion or makeup line to make people feel right at home. It's about making things cozy. And all it takes is a little thought and a little . . . presentation.

You also don't need to quit your day job to make things nice. There are so many shortcuts when things get hard. Do you want to make a homemade pie but don't have the time or even know how to make a pie? No problem—buy a Marie Callender's pie and serve that thang in a pretty dish. Do I ever cut up fresh tomatoes to make tomato sauce? No, I throw in a can of Ro-Tel (diced tomatoes with seasoning), and it tastes delicious.

Like so many important life lessons I learned from my mama, I learned taking a shortcut doesn't mean you care any less. Once, she had a big old bowl of salsa out to go with the tortilla chips, and Steve commented on how good it was. "Did you make this?" he asked.

"Yes, I did," she said.

And she did—by pouring four half-eaten jars of different salsa together.

HOME DRESSIN'

Anyone's first experience of a home is how it looks (and smells). I've lived in lots of different places, from tiny, dark rentals to big, beautiful houses. But no matter where I'm resting my head, I always make every home very, well, homey. That can be as simple as picking up flowers from the grocery store once a week and lighting a bunch of candles whenever I'm home. Those little things go such a long way.

If you want to take it up a notch, however, here are a few ideas to create a cozy, inviting environment.

SOFT ACCENTS

You can never go wrong with a lot of throw pillows and blankets. And you don't have to spend a lot of money on them. I have pillows and blankets everywhere in my house—and pretty much all of them are from Target. To keep your pillows and blankets from veering away from cozy into messy, toss them into pretty baskets that sit beside the couch.

LONG DRAPES

Curtains bring a lot of style to any room. One big mistake is cutting the drapes too short. Let them hit the ground. An even more common mistake is starting the drapes from the top of the window when they should really start from the ceiling. When you put the curtain rod at the top of the window instead of the ceiling, it visually cuts the room in half. If you start the drapes from the ceiling and let them finish at the floor, it elongates the room and is so elegant.

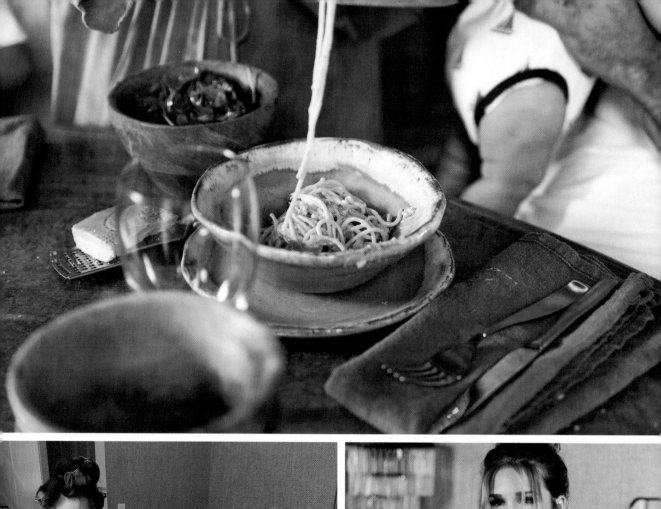
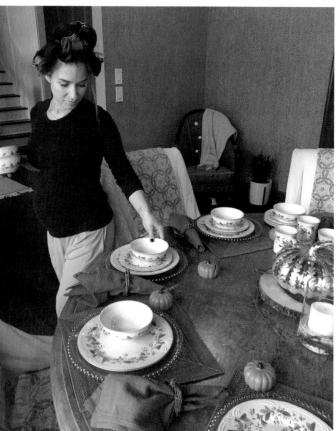
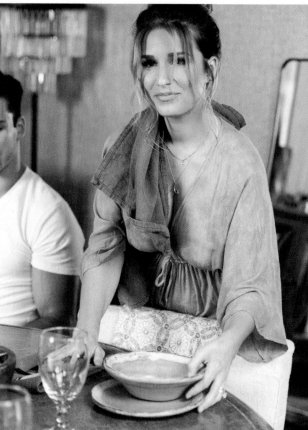

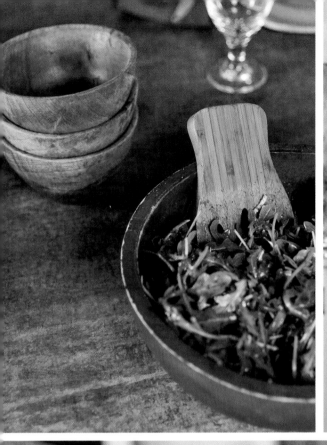
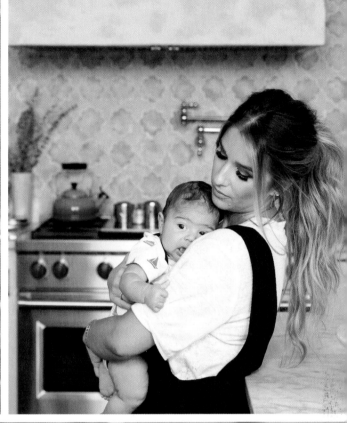
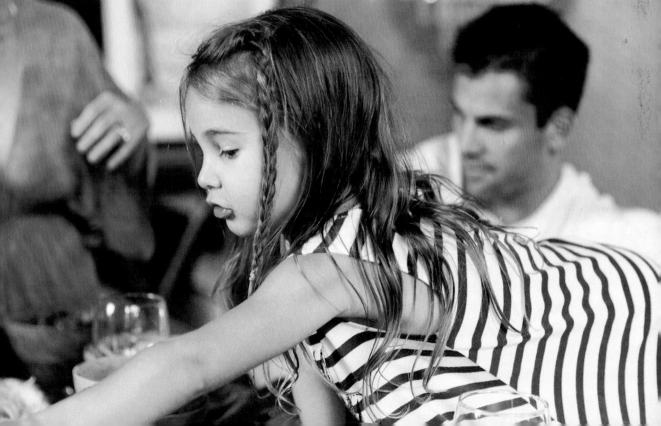

MASSIVE MIRRORS

These open up your home and make your house look bigger than it is.

FABULOUS RUGS

This is one of the easiest decorating tools. One beautiful rug can pull together an entire room and bring lots of style.

CANDLES

I'm obsessed with candles (in case you couldn't already tell). In my world, you can never have too many. Their soft lighting instantly creates a mood, and the fragrance also adds an inviting vibe.

jessie says

create a theme

When I'm decorating, I'm all about the theme. In Colorado, I dug deep into the Aspen snow lodge look with patterns and a lot of fake fur. My first house in Nashville was very southern—French country by way of Joanna Gaines. It was really beautiful and romantic. But when Eric and I moved to our current house in Nashville, I decided to switch it up again. I'm always changing my mind and my style—and right now my style's become more sleek and modern with hints of Spanish influence. (The kitchen has Spanish tiling, and I had my fireplace mortar rubbed to look like something you'd see in a gorgeous hotel in Cabo.)

I'm a mix of classic and trendy. I have elements that I'll always love—like my pillows, blankets, drapes, and photos of the babies and family everywhere. But because my favorite home decor sources and stores are always updating their style, I like to do the same.

I periodically check out what Target is up to. I think it has the best stuff. I also shop a lot at HomeGoods, Joss & Main, and even Amazon. These sites and stores can be very overwhelming. So before I shop, I look at a lot of pictures on home design websites and Pinterest and in magazines. There's this idea with decorating that you either have the eye or you don't. But with so many examples out there on the internet, I think anyone can put together their home so it's pretty.

When I find images I like—for example, a beautifully done side table for Thanksgiving—I try to emulate what people have created. I got my entire Thanksgiving and Christmas table sets off Amazon. After I found pretty table settings on Pinterest, I went to Amazon and searched for each item on the table until my table was complete. While I got it all for close to nothing, I bet most people who came over thought it was from Pottery Barn. Why throw down a lot of cash for something you use only once a year?

DECORATING WITH CHILDREN IN MIND

I haven't let my babies get in the way of having great style. I have heard from a lot of other moms that kids mess with everything. My kids don't. There are so many little things they could get into and break. I have an entire basket of messy ornaments waiting to go up on the Christmas tree that they could just terrorize. I have a glass cart in another corner with a bunch of glass bottles. But I don't worry since I know they won't fool with any of it. They're not interested.

I think the reason is that I provide them with their own toys in nearly every room. In some spaces, like the family room, they have their own tables and baskets filled with their things. Even in my living room, I keep a few drawers in a side table dedicated to their toys. It's a way to keep things clean. But they also know that when they open them up, they'll find their stuff. That's what they mess with.

The only aspect of my style I changed when I had children was eliminating very sharp edges. I swapped out a lot of my hard, pointy tables with ottomans. If you have little ones at home, do not buy hard-edged glass side tables or coffee tables. Just don't even bother with them. If you already have those pieces and aren't able to replace them, put rubber covers on the corners (we did a lot of that). I don't care if it looks pretty or not. It's better to have ugly rubber bumpers than your kid's head busted open.

THE BEDROOM

The most important thing to me in the entire house is my bed. If you're going to spend money, invest in your bed—and everything that goes with it. My mattress, which is amazing, was expensive. My sheets are also always on the pricier side. Some of my favorite sheets are actually made by Tempur-Pedic. They're the most comfortable sheets I've ever slept in in my life. This element of decorating is about more than just style. Getting a good night's sleep is essential to one's health. Every time we get in our bed, Eric and I go, "Ohhhhh yeahhhhhh." It's just the best.

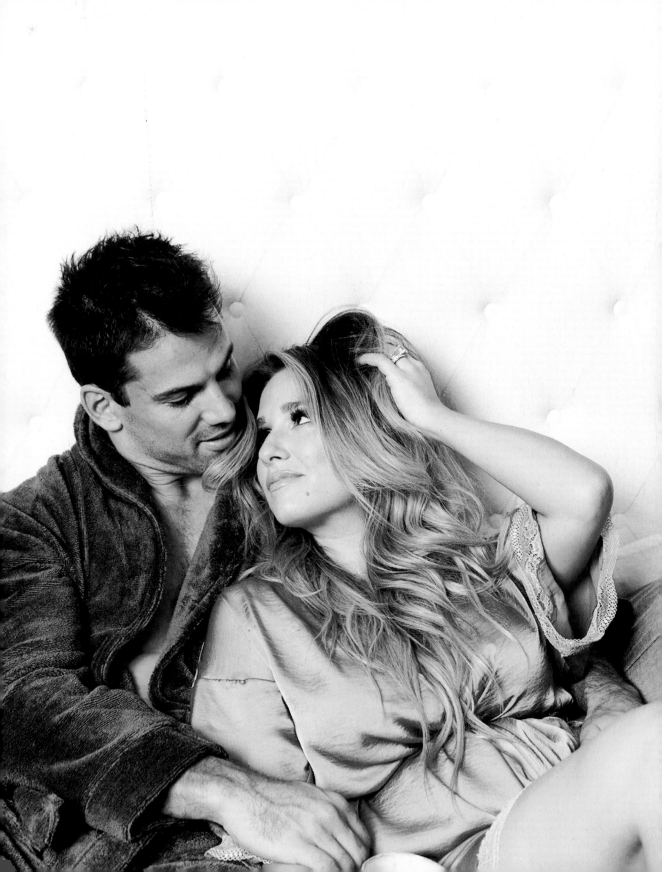

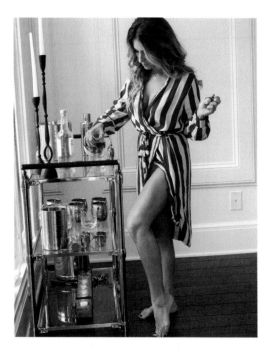

* Pretty bar carts

* Throw blankets

* Greenery (even if it's fake)

* Drapes

* Themed coffee mugs for every season (because I love coffee)

* Framed pictures of my family (I'm really terrible at getting pictures printed out and framed, so when close friends or family ask me what I want for my birthday or Christmas, I tell them to give me a framed photo. Pretty much every single picture in my house was given to me by a family member.)

HOLIDAY DECORATIONS

Starting in October with Halloween, I put up lots of decorations: pumpkins, little witches, ghosts—anything that makes it fun and gets the kids excited. To me, that's the entire point of holiday decorations—to switch it up and create a festive mood in the house. For Thanksgiving, I just take away the really Halloween-y things and am left with all the harvest decorations. For Christmas, though, I bring out the big guns. There are Christmas frames, Christmas bedspreads, stuffed Santa Clauses for the children's rooms, and sparkly or furry pillows for the living room. I cover all the staircase bannisters with garlands. And no holiday season would be complete without candles. I have a million of them.

Christmas, even the decorations, is about building traditions. When we were growing up, my mom would buy us mini–Christmas trees and put one in each of our rooms. That's where all the ornaments we made at school or church went. Every year, those ornaments kept adding up and adding up—to the point where, in high school, our personalized trees that my mom kept buying were covered in our handmade ornaments. That's a tradition I loved so much that I will carry it on with my own children.

Our main tree is still a child-centric affair. (First off, we do the fake tree, because the live ones are really messy, and if the dogs eat the pine needles, it's terrible for them.) We let the kids have fun decorating it. I think a Christmas tree looks better when it's not really put together and fancy. Again, I take a page from my own childhood by turning the tree trimming into a mini-event. When I was a kid, my mom would make hot apple cider and cookies and put on Christmas music. Then she and Steve handed the ornaments one by one to my sister, my

brother, and me. I loved the ritual—and do it with my own kids, who
love it just as much.

ORGANIZATION

My family calls me Messica Jessica, because I'm a very messy person.
I don't pretend to be organized, because I'm not and never will be. My
brain just doesn't work that way. Eric is the neat freak. He cleans. I don't.
I see it as part of the deal. As I always say to him, "When it comes to
looking good, making good food, and cleaning, I can only do two out of
three. What are the two most important to you?" So he cleans.

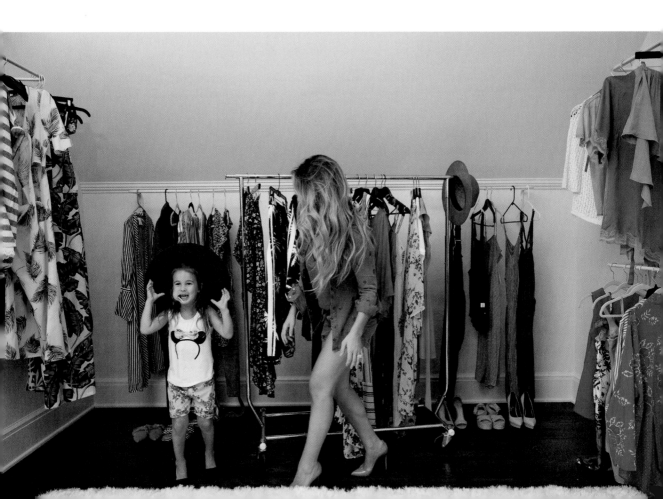

But there does come a time (usually when you have kids) when you need a certain level of organization to function. In the kitchen, I used to have half-open bags of flour and sugar and crap everywhere. My spices were all over the place. And don't even get me started about my closet. With three small children and a full-time career, the last thing I want to do is organize the house. Some folks are just born with certain talents. I don't run that way and I never will. But I have other skills. So I ask friends who do work that way to come over and help me organize my closet and bathroom. I repay the favor with something I'm good at, like doing their hair or makeup for an event. One girlfriend created a system for me that I try to follow, but sometimes I just need her to come back and do a good

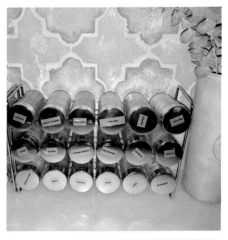

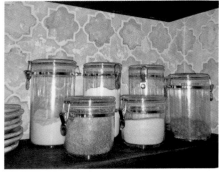

cleaning out. In return, she borrows clothes from my closet or I get her ready for an event. It's not only a great way to keep my life organized, but sharing our gifts with each other is also a wonderful expression of our friendship.

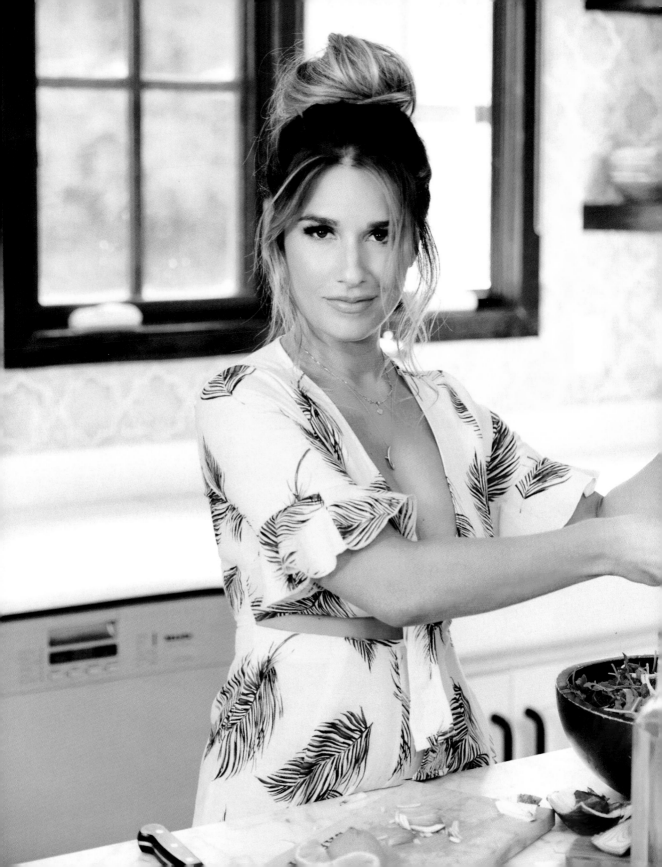

in the kitchen

Cooking should be fun and festive. There is something about it that sets the tone in the house. Food is hugely important to me and always has been since I was little. I was taught by my mama that everything is about presentation and not to ever skimp on that. Now, I know it can't be that way every time. There are nights when I have thirty minutes to make something (those recipes are here too). But on the nights when there is no rush, make it fabulous and festive. It's all about enjoying the little moments in life. Some of my best memories are of dancing to sexy music in the kitchen while having a glass of wine or iced tea, enjoying my husband's company, and feeding the babies samples of food, like when I would put Viv on the counter, sneaking kisses and tastes in between the cooking. Creating delicious meals for the ones I love is one of my favorite things to do. That's why I made sure I added some of my favorite tips and recipes, so you can share this with your family too.

HOME GATHERINGS

One day a girlfriend popped over for a visit, so I threw together what I always do: cheese, olives, crackers, some cut-up veggies, and honey on a wooden tray. My friend surveyed the pretty tray of food, popped an olive in her mouth, and said, "How do you always put out this kind of spread? I could never do all this."

"Yes, you could. This is nothing. This took me no time. You just think it did, but it didn't."

My friend didn't believe me, but it's true. It's not false modesty. When I entertain at home, it sure looks pretty (and tastes good), but there's nothing hard about it. Again, it's all about presentation. My little secret is . . . cutting boards and platters. I'm serious! I have so many of those things in all shapes, sizes, and materials. And most of them are not expensive. One of my favorites cost me ten dollars from Target, and

jessie says

when you have time to enjoy cooking . . .

* Light some candles
* Put out a wooden platter with a few appetizers, such as some cheese with a little honey and crackers
* Play some bossa nova or French jazz
* Pour some vino for you and your man

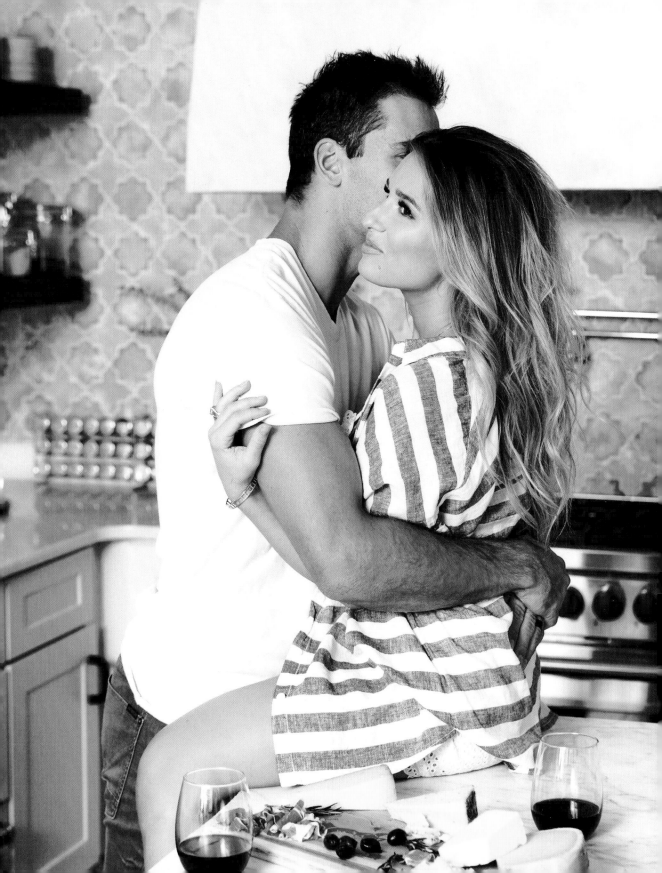

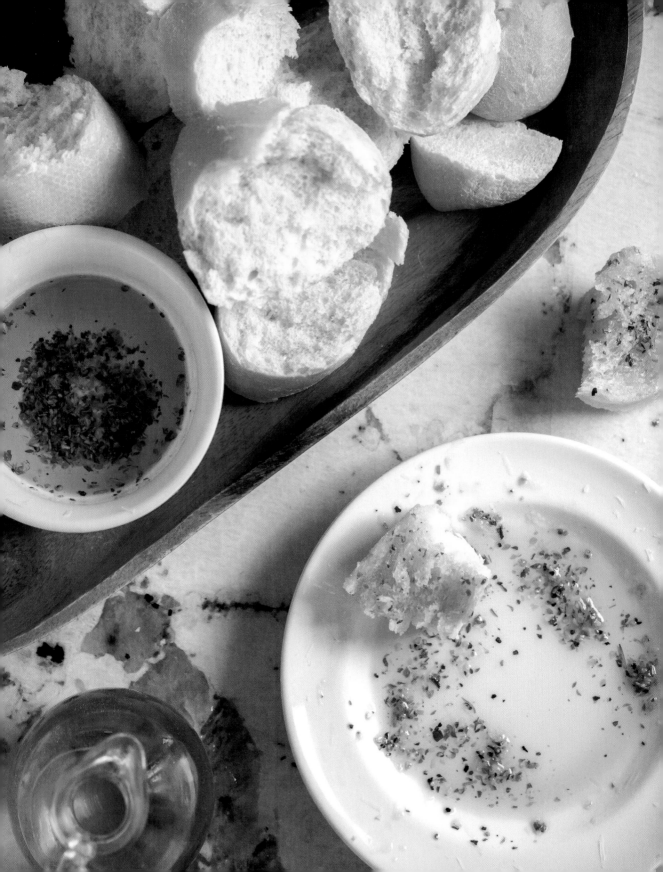

destin dipping oil

MAKES 1 CUP DIPPING OIL

1 cup extra virgin olive oil

½ tablespoon dried basil

1 tablespoon garlic powder

1 tablespoon chili flakes

½ teaspoon salt

½ teaspoon black pepper

2 cloves garlic, minced

Juice of ½ lemon

Parmesan, to taste

1 loaf French bread

My parents used to take us to Destin, Florida, when we were kids. Some of my happiest memories as a child were during those trips with my family. We didn't have a lot of money, but my parents never let that get in the way of having fun. We would pack up the car and drive six hours from Georgia to Florida with our golden retriever, Talon, lying across the laps of my brother, my sister, and me. Sharing one hotel room, my siblings and I slept on some blankets on the floor and called it an adventure! I was so grateful I never knew that we were doing it on such little cash. Because it was so costly, we typically didn't eat out the whole week. (My mom would get all the groceries from a commissary.) Once during the week, we went out to dinner at this little Italian pizza place. It was a real treat, and the best part about it was this addictive dipping oil that came with the French bread. I never learned the exact recipe, but I have to say my take on it is pretty darn close! So now every time I make this dipping oil, I think about those good times in Destin.

Preheat the oven to 350°F.

In a small bowl, whisk together the olive oil, basil, garlic powder, chili flakes, salt, pepper, and garlic. Squeeze some lemon juice in and mix. Sprinkle freshly grated Parmesan cheese over the surface of the mixture.

Throw the loaf of French bread in the oven for 8 minutes. Remove the loaf and place it on a cutting board, slice up the warm bread, and put it in a white serving bowl. Serve alongside the dipping oil and watch it all disappear.

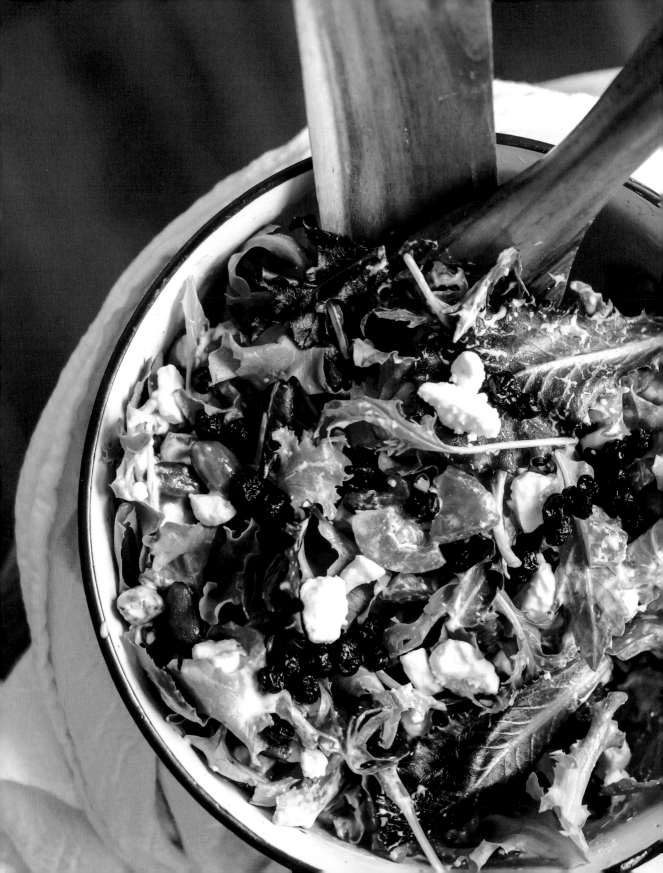

bay salad

FOR THE DRESSING

¼ cup plain yogurt

¼ cup Meyer lemon juice

½ cup extra virgin olive oil

¼ cup honey

Salt, to taste

Black pepper, to taste

FOR THE SALAD

One 5-ounce bag mixed greens

1 cup dried blueberries

1 cup honey-roasted almonds

1 cup feta cheese

1 cup diced tomatoes

This salad is amazing alone, but throwing some grilled shrimp over it makes it even more delicious.

In a small bowl, whisk together the dressing ingredients until combined and set aside. In a salad bowl, assemble the salad ingredients. Add the dressing, toss to mix, and season with salt and pepper to taste.

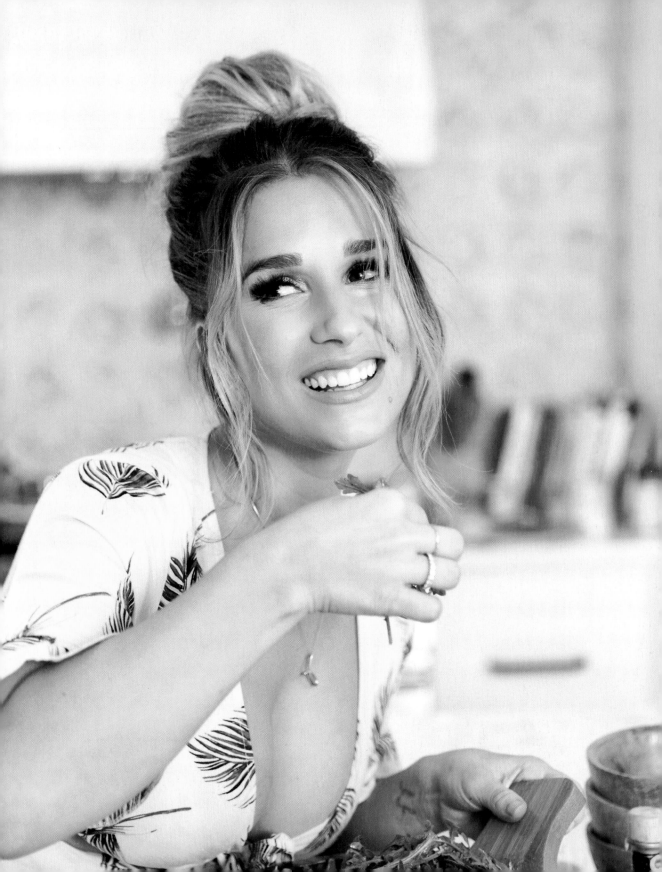

watermelon feta salad

**MAKES 5 TO 6 SERVINGS
AS A SIDE DISH, 3 TO 5 AS
A MAIN ENTRÉE**

This salad is gorgeous and colorful and perfect for summer. I will make this as an appetizer or sometimes grill some chicken and throw it on top.

FOR THE DRESSING

¼ cup extra virgin olive oil

2 tablespoons sherry vinegar or red wine vinegar

Juice of ½ lemon

1 teaspoon Truvia sweetener

Garlic powder, to taste

Salt, to taste

Black pepper, to taste

FOR THE SALAD

5 ounces arugula

3½ ounces crumbled feta cheese

½ medium red onion, sliced thin

Several mint leaves, torn up

2 cups watermelon, cubed

Garlic powder, to taste (yes, more garlic powder—I put it on everything!)

In a small bowl, whisk together the dressing ingredients until combined and set aside. In a salad bowl, assemble the salad ingredients. Add the dressing, toss to mix, and season with salt and pepper to taste.

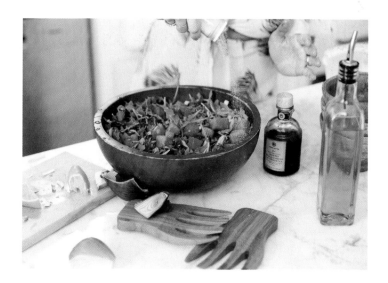

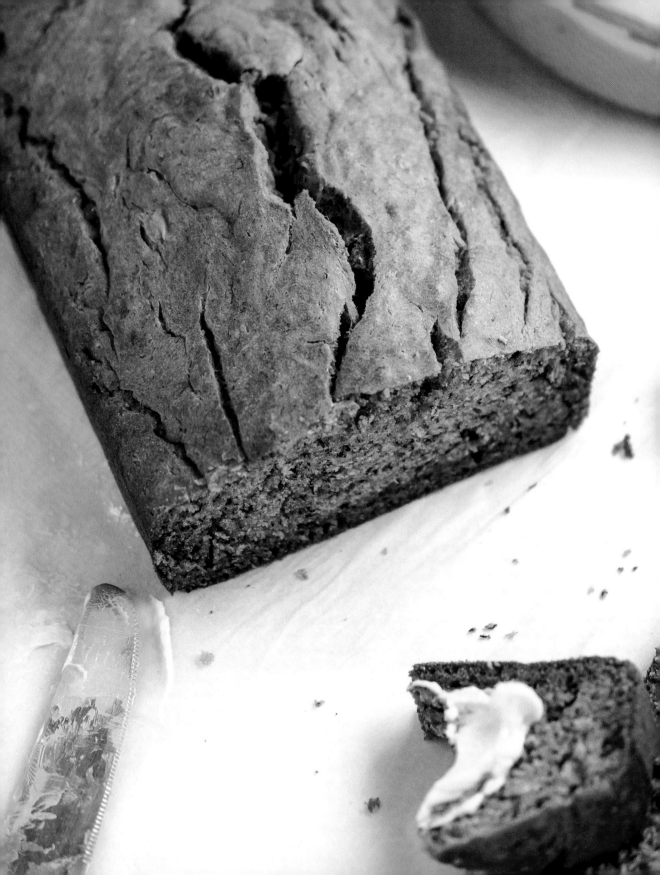

banana bread

MAKES 1 LOAF

Butter, for the loaf pan

3 ripe bananas, mashed

2 eggs

¼ cup brown sugar

1 teaspoon vanilla

1 stick unsalted butter

¾ teaspoon cinnamon

2 teaspoons maple syrup

1½ cups all-purpose flour

1 teaspoon baking soda

½ teaspoon pink Himalayan salt

Banana bread is a must in our house. I have been making this for years, and every time I do, it ends up gone within hours. Last time my brother caught wind that I was baking it, and he came over to the house to make sure I made him an extra loaf to bring home. I love this for breakfast in the morning with warm butter and a nice hot cup of coffee.

Preheat the oven to 350°F. Butter an 8½-x-4½-inch loaf pan and set aside.

In a large bowl, combine the bananas, eggs, brown sugar, vanilla, butter, cinnamon, and maple syrup. In a separate bowl, combine the flour, baking soda, and salt.

Add the dry flour mixture to the banana mixture. Combine and pour into the loaf pan. Bake for 50 minutes or until a toothpick inserted into the center comes out cleanly.

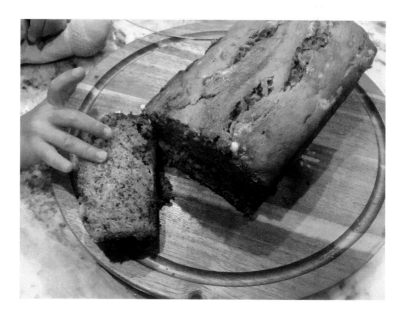

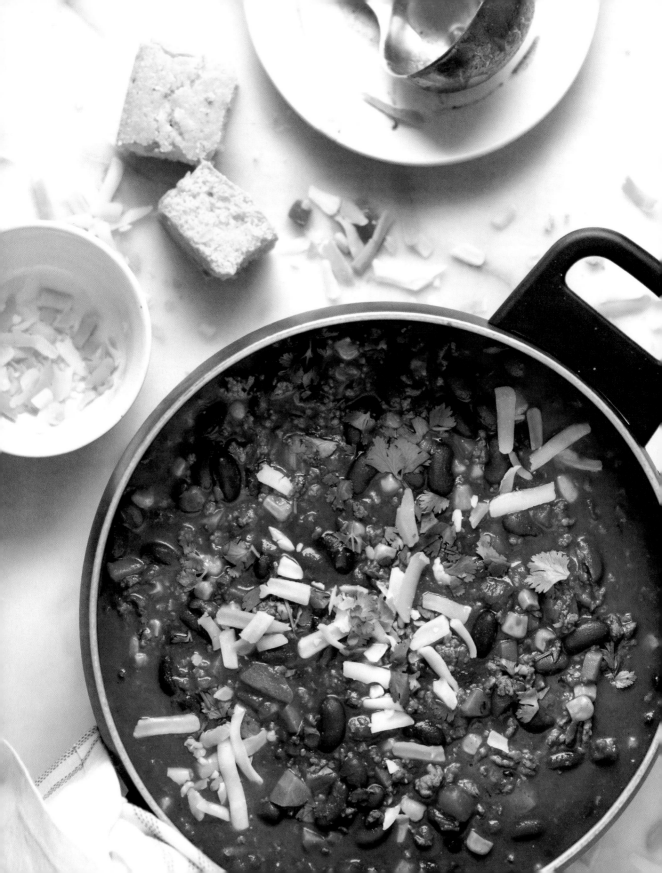

jessie's sexy chili

MAKES 6 TO 8 SERVINGS

2 tablespoons olive oil

2 cloves garlic, chopped

3 carrots, chopped

1 medium yellow or white onion, chopped

1 pound ground beef

1 10-ounce can of Ro-Tel Mild Seasoned Diced Tomatoes & Green Chilies

3 15-ounce cans kidney beans, drained and rinsed

½ 16-ounce bag frozen white corn

1 15-ounce can vegetarian chili

½ 15-ounce can tomato sauce

2 tablespoons chili powder

1 teaspoon cumin

1 tablespoon garlic powder

Salt, to taste

Black pepper, to taste

Tony Chachere's Original Creole Seasoning (optional, if you want to spice it up)

Cheddar cheese, grated to serve

Cornbread, to serve

Tortilla chips, to serve

I love chili and always have. I have about six or seven different versions, but this is Eric's favorite. I know because when I make it for him he gives me lovey sexy eyes with every bite.

Men love hearty, meaty meals, and this is a way to make them very happy. This is perfect for game days, cold winter nights, or just when you want some darn chili! I always have these ingredients on hand, because in addition to tasting great, it's one of the easiest meals to make.

In a large pot over medium heat, drizzle in the olive oil. Add the garlic and sauté until it becomes fragrant. Add the carrots and onion. When they start to soften (and smell amazing), add the ground beef. When the meat is cooked, add the Ro-Tel, kidney beans, corn, vegetarian chili, and tomato sauce. Combine and cook for 5 minutes, then add the chili powder, cumin, and garlic powder, and season to taste. Mix, cover, and turn the heat to low until you are ready to eat.

To serve, smother each bowl of chili in cheese and set out with a side of cornbread. Or put out tortilla chips to dip into the chili and then watch your man's eyes stare at you in that sexy way with every bite.

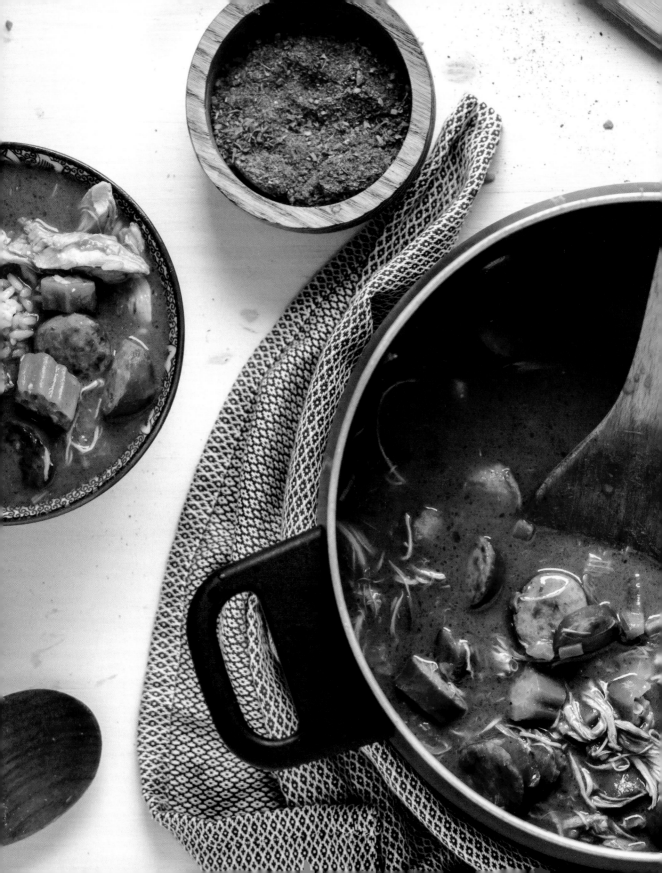

chicken and sausage gumbo

MAKES 10 SERVINGS

FOR THE ROUX

1 cup all-purpose flour

Salt, to taste

Black pepper, to taste

Tony Chachere's Original Creole Seasoning, to taste

1 cup olive or canola oil

1 medium yellow onion, chopped

1 cup celery, chopped

1 green bell pepper, chopped

4 cloves garlic, minced

2 quarts chicken stock

3 cups cooked shredded chicken

1 package smoked sausage, sliced and cooked

Cayenne, to taste

Filé, to taste

3 cups frozen sliced okra

3 green onions, chopped

White rice, to serve

Cajun food will always have a special place in my heart because it was my first love—well, first love of food. In Louisiana, where my mom was born and raised, you can get delicious po-boys at drive-throughs and fresh crawfish (when in season) anywhere. In fact, some of the best red beans and rice I've ever had was at a Louisiana gas station. This recipe is straight from a cookbook my mama made for me when I got married to Eric. This page, covered in grease and oil, is by far the dirtiest page in the book, because gumbo is one of my favorite meals to eat and to make. This version is so good it won a contest on Rachael Ray, where Eric and I competed against two other couples to see who could make the best dish!

Make the roux: In a heavy Dutch oven over medium heat, add the flour and seasoning and pour in the oil, continuously stirring with a wooden spoon until the mixture turns a rich dark brown. Be careful not to burn the mixture. Do not leave the pot or the spoon unattended, or you might have to start again.

To the roux, add the onion, celery, and bell pepper. Cook until soft. Add the garlic, chicken stock, shredded chicken, sausage, cayenne, and filé. Simmer on low heat for at least 2 hours. Add the okra, green onions, and additional seasonings to taste. Keep on low heat all day until ready to eat. Serve over white rice.

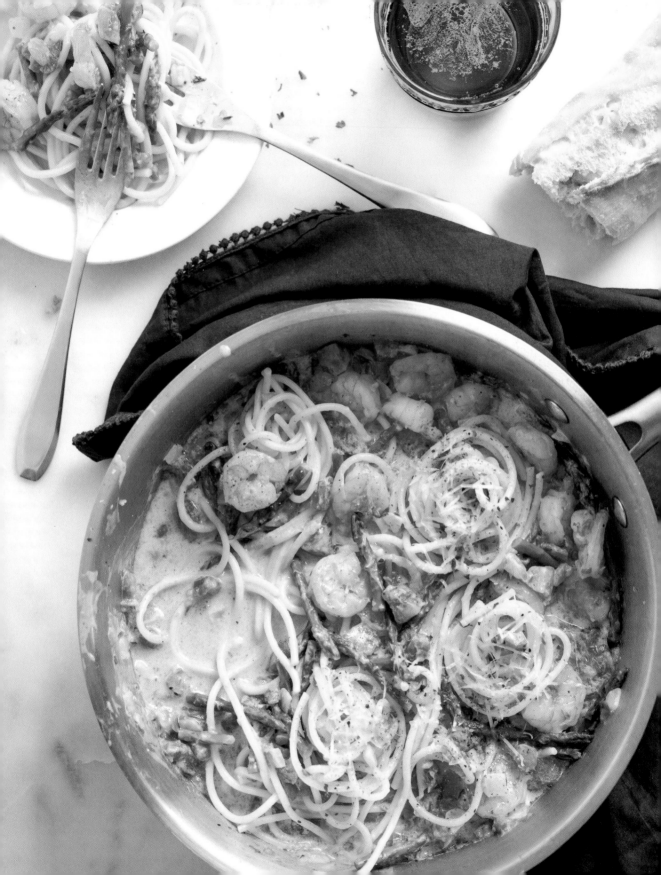

mama's cajun shrimp pasta

MAKES 4 TO 6 SERVINGS

1 pound pasta of choice

3 tablespoons butter

¼ cup yellow onion, diced

1 bunch asparagus, trimmed and cut on a diagonal in inch-long pieces

1 pound medium shrimp, peeled and deveined

Salt, to taste

Black pepper, to taste

Slap Ya Mama Original Blend Cajun Seasoning, to taste

1 10-oz can Ro-Tel Mild Seasoned Diced Tomatoes & Green Chilies

½ cup half-and-half

Parmesan cheese, to serve

I grew up on Cajun food, the best food in the world! My whole family comes from Louisiana, which always feels like home to me: the music, the people, the landscape. But out of everything, it's the food that touches me the deepest. I learned these recipes from my mama, who learned them from her mama, who learned them from my Sicilian great-grandmother.

Mama's Cajun Shrimp Pasta has been a mega-hit for years! When you put this together people will think you are a fancy chef, because the presentation is beautiful and the flavors are ridiculously good. My mom invented this recipe when we were kids, and I decided to share it with the world on The Chew. *It was a secret recipe, but Mama was a trooper about it. I then made her put it on her blog because people kept begging for this incredible dish!*

Cook the pasta according to the package instructions and drain. Set aside.

In a skillet over medium heat, melt the butter. Add the onion and sauté for about 2 minutes. Add the asparagus and sauté for 3 minutes. Add the shrimp and cook for 4 minutes. Season with salt, pepper, and Slap Ya Mama Cajun Seasoning. Pour in the Ro-Tel and half-and-half and simmer over low heat for 5 minutes. Remove from the heat and pour over the pasta. Toss to coat the pasta thoroughly, sprinkle with Parmesan cheese, and serve immediately.

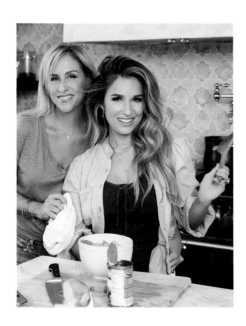

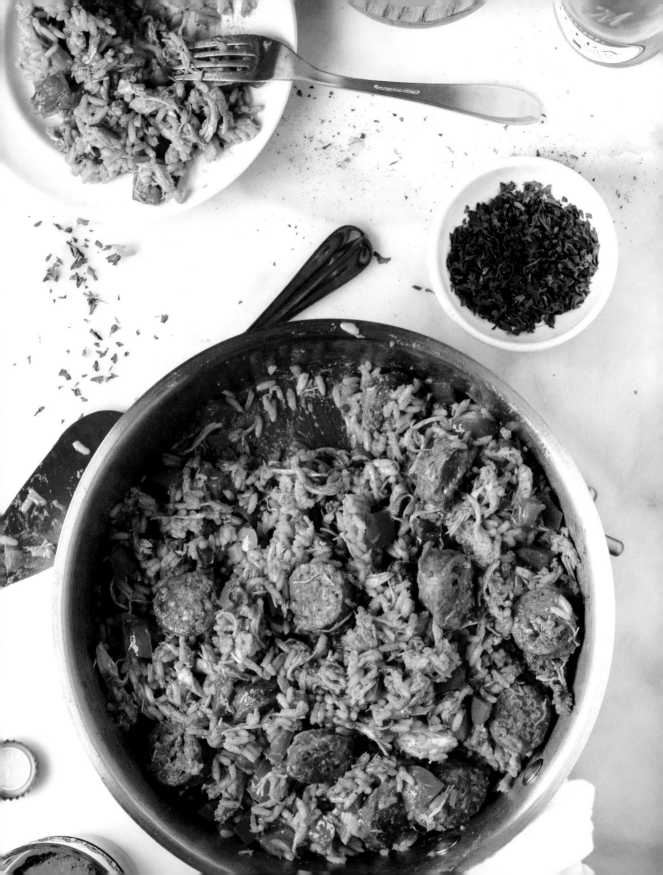

jambalaya

MAKES 6 SERVINGS

2 tablespoons olive oil

12 ounces Polska Kielbasa sausage (pork, beef, or turkey), cut into bite-size pieces

1 rotisserie chicken, meat removed and shredded with a fork

½ medium yellow onion, chopped

½ red bell pepper, chopped

½ green bell pepper, chopped

½ yellow bell pepper, chopped

1 box Zatarain's Jambalaya Mix

Salt, to taste

Black pepper, to taste

Tony Chachere's Original Creole Seasoning, to taste

This is the first thing I ever learned to cook! It was my first time cooking alone in a kitchen and I was so nervous! I was so overwhelmed with the sausage sizzling, the water boiling, and the vegetables needing chopping. But I have now perfected this easy recipe, which helped sealed the deal with Eric during our first weekend together in Nashville. (My sister also made this for her husband, Anthony, to seal the deal!)

Drizzle 1 tablespoon olive oil in a pan, add cut-up sausage and sauté over medium-high heat for about 5 minutes. Add the chicken meat and continue sautéing until the sausage is cooked all the way through, about 5 additional minutes.

In a separate pan, drizzle the remaining olive oil and add the onion and peppers, cooking over medium-high heat until they get soft and fragrant, about 10 minutes.

Follow the directions on the box to make the Zatarain's Jambalaya Mix.

Add the cooked sausage-chicken combo and cooked onion and peppers to the pot of rice.

Add salt, pepper, garlic powder, and Tony seasoning to taste. Stir, and then turn your heat down to low and cover the pot. Set a timer for 20 minutes, stirring occasionally, and it's done!

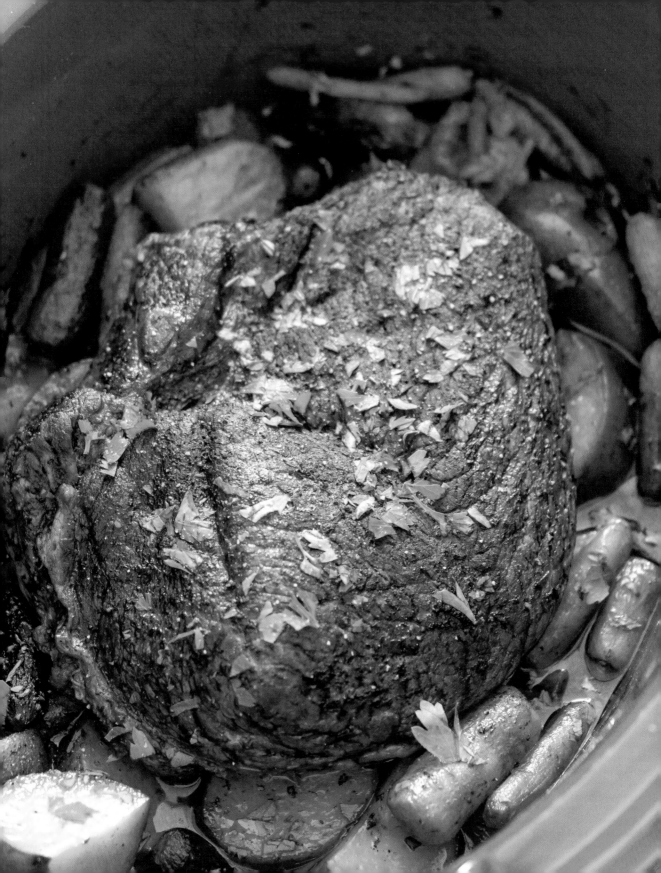

hearty slow-cooker pot roast

MAKES 8 SERVINGS

Equipment: Crock-Pot

2 medium yellow onions, sliced

1 4-pound rump roast (you can vary the size depending on how many people you want to serve; a general rule of thumb is a half pound per serving)

Salt, to taste

Black pepper, to taste

Olive oil, for the pan and to drizzle

1 12-ounce bag baby carrots

1 2-pound sack Yukon Gold potatoes (cut in halves or quarters, if large)

Garlic powder, to taste

Tony Chachere's Original Creole Seasoning, to taste

Rice, to serve

Dinner rolls, to serve

Cinnamon butter, to serve

This is one of the first meals I ever taught myself how to make. Eric and I had just moved in together in Colorado, and I was in a hurry to start learning how to cook for him. I have never enjoyed eating out as much as I enjoy a home-cooked meal. I blame my mother and the other Italian women in my family. They are such incredible cooks that I somehow got the idea that all food was that fabulous.

I wanted to make sure I gave the same to my new love and first live-in boyfriend. I love all kinds of foods—Cajun, Italian, and good ole meat and potatoes. Eric is a midwestern guy, and I wanted to make my Yankee boyfriend proud that his southern girlfriend could whip up some meat and potatoes too.

Okay, back to the recipe. I did a lot of research on the best way to make this roast, and after I got the gist I created this recipe. Eric loves this meal, which I have been making for the last seven years. It's perfect for those days when you know you will be swamped or gone and there won't be time to make dinner when you finally get home. You prep it first thing in the morning, and it cooks all day.

Turn your Crock-Pot on the high setting and set the timer for 7 hours. Add the onions.

Sprinkle the roast with salt and pepper. In a pan over medium-high heat, heat up the olive oil. Add the roast and brown on both sides. Place the roast in the Crock-Pot. Throw the carrots and potatoes on top of that. Drizzle with some more olive oil and season with garlic powder, Tony seasoning, salt, and pepper. Put the lid on top and wait for the whole house to fill up with that hearty smell. When it is finished, serve over rice and with warm rolls and cinnamon butter.

sea bass meal

MAKES 4 SERVINGS

FOR THE CREAM SAUCE

2 tablespoons butter

1 clove garlic, chopped

2 tablespoons yellow onion, chopped

½ cup heavy whipping cream

1 tablespoon vanilla

Salt, to taste

Black pepper, to taste

Pinch of sugar

Pinch of paprika

FOR THE FISH

4 4-ounce wild-caught sea bass fillets

Tony Chachere's Original Creole Seasoning, to taste

Salt, to taste

Black pepper, to taste

Olive oil, for the sheet pan

FOR THE CREAMED CAULIFLOWER

½ cup water

1 16-ounce bag of pre-riced cauliflower (frozen or fresh)

Olive oil, to drizzle

2 tablespoons butter

½ teaspoon dried thyme

3 tablespoons cream

Salt, to taste

Black pepper, to taste

I had this exact meal at the wedding of one of Eric's best friends, which I attended when I was pregnant with Forrest. It was so delicious that I was craving it when I got back home. So, remembering the flavors, I made up my own version of the dish—and Eric told me it's one of the best things I've ever made.

Make the cream sauce: In a saucepot over medium heat, melt the butter. Add the garlic and onion and cook until softened. Add the remaining cream sauce ingredients and stir over medium heat. Once combined, turn the heat to low and cover until the fish and cauliflower are ready.

Make the fish: Preheat the oven to 375°F. Sprinkle the sea bass fillets all over with Tony seasoning, salt, and pepper. Place the fillets on an oiled sheet pan and put in the oven. Bake for 15 to 20 minutes or until the fish turns golden brown and starts flaking.

Make the creamed cauliflower: In a small pot, bring the water to a boil. Throw in the bag of riced cauliflower, drizzle with olive oil, and let cook for 2 minutes. Add the remaining ingredients and season with salt and pepper. Stir for another 3 minutes. Transfer the cauliflower to a heatproof bowl and carefully puree with a hand blender, or transfer to the jar of a standing blender and puree. Return the mixture to the pot and keep covered over low heat until ready to serve.

Make the roasted tri-color baby carrots: Preheat the oven to 375°F. Lay the baby carrots out on a flat sheet pan. Drizzle with enough olive oil, garlic powder, salt, and pepper to coat thoroughly. Cook until they are roasted,

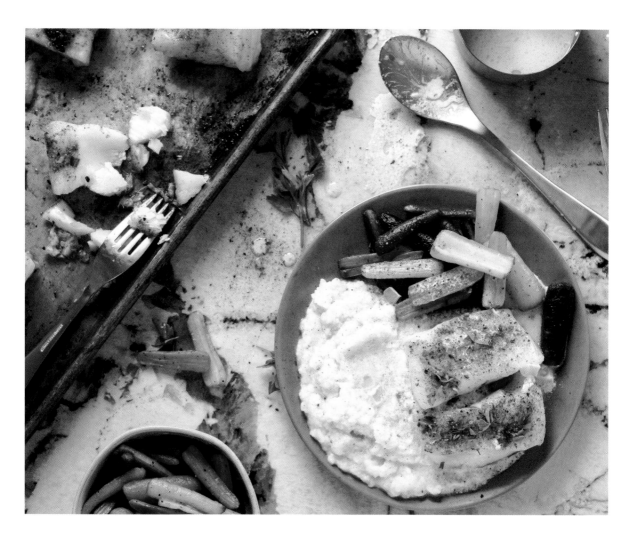

**1 12-ounce bag of tri-color
baby carrots**

Olive oil

Garlic powder, to taste

Salt, to taste

Black pepper, to taste

Parsley, to garnish

about 20 minutes. You can begin roasting while the fish is cooking, and if they aren't crispy enough when the fish comes out, turn the oven to 400°F until they are done.

To serve: Place the fish on top of the creamed cauliflower and drizzle the cream sauce over both. Garnish with parsley and serve with the roasted carrots on the side.

chicken fit-chiladas

1 teaspoon olive oil, plus more for greasing baking dish

2 garlic cloves, minced

1 cup chopped onion

2½ cups shredded chicken from a rotisserie chicken

Salt, to taste

2 tablespoons fresh cilantro

1 teaspoon cumin

1 teaspoon oregano

2 teaspoons chili powder

1 cup canned tomato sauce

½ cup chicken broth

1 can pinto beans, rinsed

Black pepper, to taste

1 teaspoon garlic powder, or more if you want

Low-carb wheat flour tortillas (I love Trader Joe's brand)

Enchilada sauce (recipe follows)

2 cups Mexican cheese

Light sour cream

Handful of chopped green onions and cilantro for garnish

I have to say that Mexican food is one of my favorite things to eat. I love all the flavors and spices. Any time I am in Mexico I eat as much as I possibly can. I will also write things down in my phone that I fell in love with so I can go back home and try to make them for my family. One dish I devour is enchiladas. While I was trying to lose weight after Bubby was born, I still wanted to enjoy my meals and feel full. So I did my research and found that enchiladas can actually be an amazing low-calorie meal for those watching their figure. These filling and delicious enchiladas are under 200 calories each!

Preheat the oven to 400°F. Drizzle olive oil in a glass baking dish until the whole thing is greased.

Heat the olive oil in a medium skillet over medium-high heat. Sauté the garlic and onion on low until soft, about 2 minutes. Add the chicken, salt, cilantro, cumin, oregano, chili powder, tomato sauce, chicken broth, and pinto beans and cook about 5 minutes. Remove from heat. Put ½ cup of chicken mixture into each tortilla, roll it, and place it in the prepared baking dish with the fold facing down. Pour the enchilada sauce over the enchiladas, smothering them. Then top with cheese. Bake for 20 minutes, or until all the cheese is melted. Top with sour cream and garnish with green onions and cilantro.

enchilada sauce

½ teaspoon olive oil

2 garlic cloves, minced

1 cup reduced-sodium chicken broth

1½ cups canned tomato sauce

2 chipotle chilies in adobo sauce, chopped

1 chili powder (or more to taste)

1 teaspoon garlic powder

1 teaspoon ground cumin

Salt, to taste

Black pepper, to taste

If you don't have time to make this, store-bought will be just fine!

Heat a saucepan over medium heat, then add the oil and garlic and sauté until golden, about 1 minute. Add the chicken broth, tomato sauce, chilies, chili powder, garlic powder, cumin, salt, and pepper. Bring the mixture to a boil, then reduce the heat to low and simmer, uncovered, for 4 minutes. Set aside until ready to use.

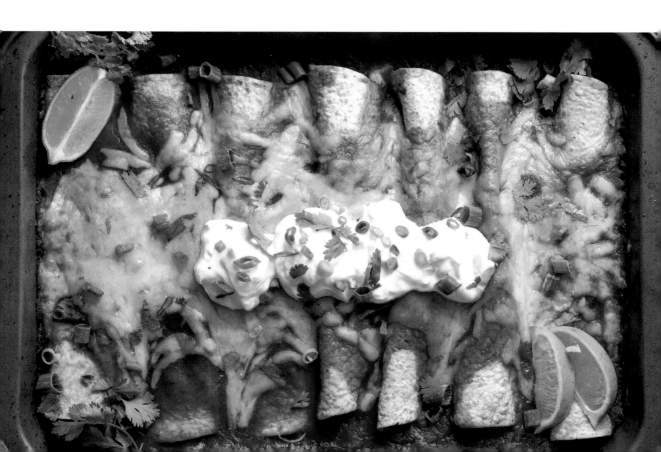

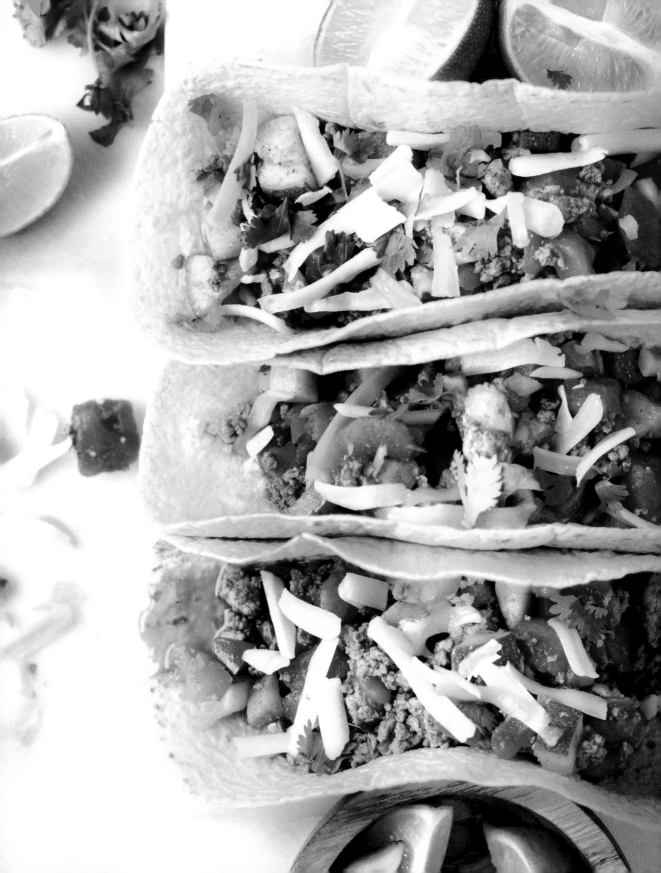

ground chicken and zucchini tacos

MAKES 10 TACOS

1 tablespoon olive oil, plus more as needed

2 zucchinis, chopped

¼ yellow onion, chopped

¼ red bell pepper, chopped

1 pound ground chicken

1 tablespoon cumin

½ tablespoon paprika

1 tablespoon chili powder

1 tablespoon garlic powder, plus more to taste

Salt, to taste

Black pepper, to taste

1 14.5-ounce can diced tomatoes

½ cup chicken broth

10 whole-wheat tortillas

Low-fat Mexican cheese, shredded for serving

We love tacos in our house and have them almost weekly. Eric got tired of having the same style of tacos all the time, so one day I decided to switch it up and use some zucchini and ground chicken I had just bought. This taco recipe was invented, and Eric looked at me with a full mouth and taco juice dripping from his chin, and said, "Add this to the weekly menu."

Drizzle the olive oil in a pan and sauté zucchini over medium-high heat for 5 minutes. Then throw in the onion and bell pepper and continue cooking until they are soft and fragrant, about 10 minutes. Season the ground chicken with the cumin, paprika, chili powder, and garlic powder. In a separate pan, brown the ground chicken. Add a little bit of olive oil so it doesn't dry out. After the chicken is cooked, about 10 minutes, add it to the vegetable mix. Season with salt, pepper, and additional garlic powder if desired. Then add the tomatoes and chicken broth

Preheat the oven to 350°F. In a separate bowl, combine a little bit of olive oil with salt and paint your tortillas with the mixture on both sides. Place the tortillas on a baking sheet in the oven for 2 to 5 minutes to heat them up. Put the ground chicken mixture in the tortillas and serve with cheese.

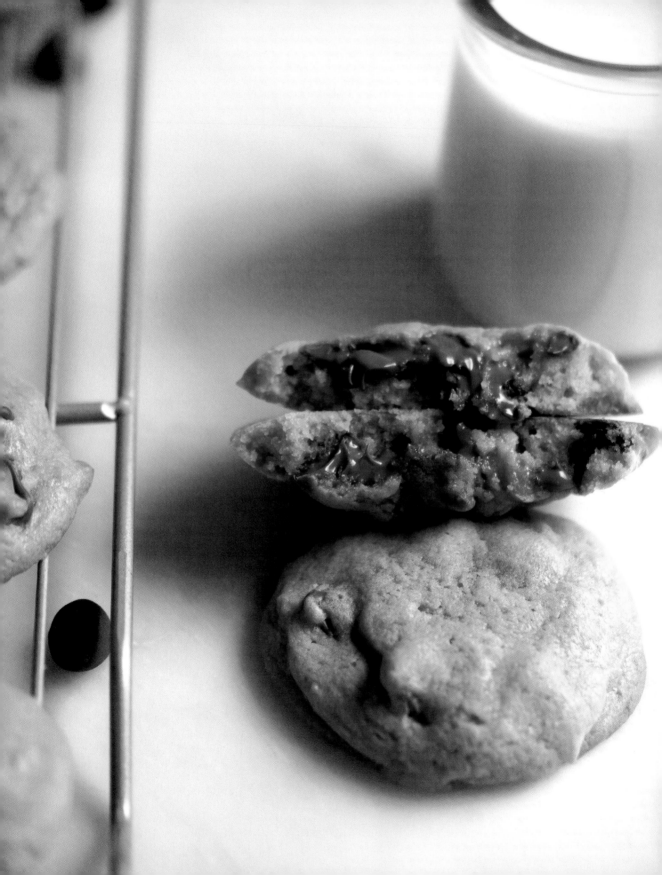

chocolate chip cookies

MAKES 3 DOZEN COOKIES

1 cup grass-fed butter, softened, plus more for greasing cookie sheet

2½ cups flour

1 teaspoon baking soda

1 teaspoon salt

½ cup cane sugar

1 cup light brown sugar

1 teaspoon pink Himalayan salt

2 teaspoons vanilla extract

2 large eggs

2 cups semisweet chocolate chips

Chocolate chip cookies are my favorite dessert in the whole entire world. Everyone knows it: my friends, my family, even my fans. They all know. So I consider myself a chocolate chip cookie connoisseur. Throughout the years I have researched and tried many different recipes until I finally came up with one that my family and I fell in love with. The Himalayan salt and the two teaspoons of vanilla are what makes these special.

Preheat the oven to 375°F. Prepare a cookie sheet by rubbing it with butter.

Combine flour, baking soda, and salt in small bowl. Beat butter, sugar, brown sugar, salt, and vanilla extract in a large mixing bowl until creamy. Add eggs, one at a time, beating well after each addition. Pour slowly into the flour mixture. Next, throw in the chocolate chips. After scooping the dough onto a cookie sheet, bake for about 10 minutes, or until golden brown. Cool on baking sheets for a couple of minutes, but not so long that the cookies continue to bake. Place the cookies on a pretty platter and enjoy!

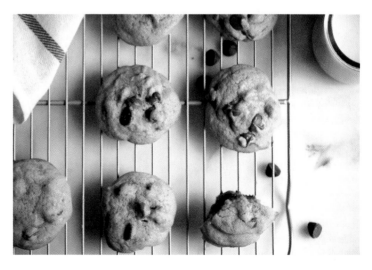

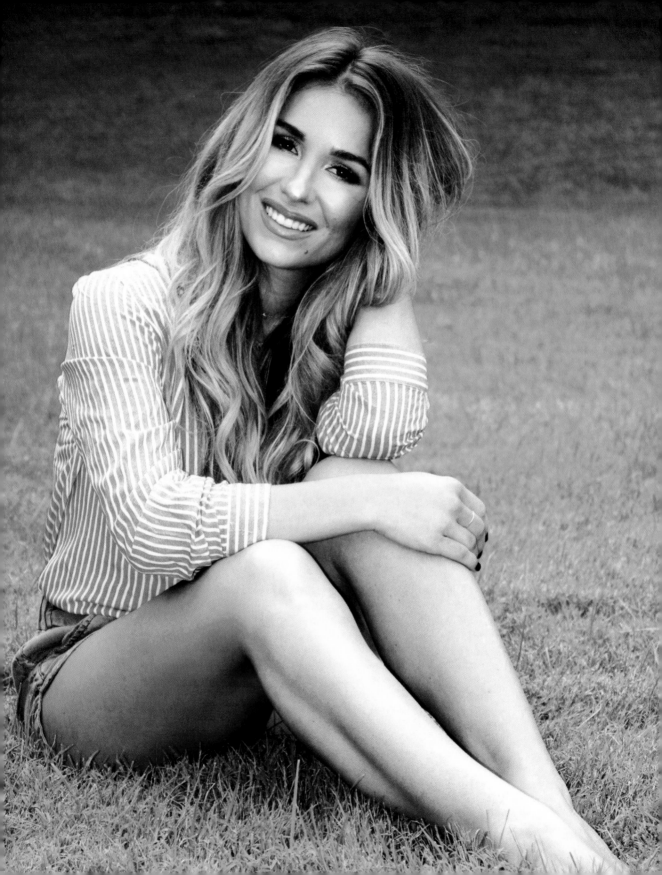

beauty is as beauty does

I'm pretty hands-on with my own beauty, especially since becoming a mom. Lots of women assume that because I'm an entertainer, I go to masseuses, trainers, stylists, manicurists, and hairdressers all day long. They're out of their damn minds. With three kids, I can barely squeeze in fifteen minutes to blow-dry my hair after a bath.

In fact, I sometimes highlight my own hair, because I feel bad leaving the kids for three hours. Sound familiar? Most women feel this way. Still, there are ways to primp without having to leave the house for hours at the spa or salon.

I love beauty: playing around with the newest products and styles, and learning new tricks and tips on how to feel beautiful and confident. If I were not in the entertainment world, I would

* False eyelashes and glue. If you can't afford to get them professionally done, these are great. They just take a little practice.

* Revlon Frost & Glow highlighting kit. Because I'm very particular about my hair color, I did it myself for years. Even now if I can't get to the salon or want to tweak something, I just do it myself!

* L'Oréal Paris Sublime Bronze Tinted Self-Tanning Lotion

* Mane 'n Tail shampoo and conditioner. I swear by this brand and have for years. It costs next to nothing, and you get massive jugs of it.

* L'Oréal Paris Voluminous Original Mascara

have done something in hair and makeup right there with my best friend, Jessica. What I've found from experimenting all these years is that you *can* do beauty on a budget, and it's worth an investment of time.

I'm always encouraging women who don't think they have the time or money to look good to stop thinking that way. Like I said before, if your hair and makeup look great, everything else looks better. I do believe that. That doesn't mean, however, you have to be dolled up all the time. That's unrealistic and exhausting. Putting yourself together, just a little bit, can make the world of difference in how you feel. I always say to Eric, "Do you want me to look good today? 'Cause if you do, I need you to watch the kids for twenty minutes. If not, this is what you get."

I don't think Eric really cares if I wear any makeup or not, but he gets that I feel better when I get a little time to myself, even if it's just to put on moisturizer and illuminator and to fix my hair. (I always have eyelash extensions. I get them done regularly. It might seem high maintenance, but it's actually low maintenance, because I wake up and they're just there. I don't have to do anything. It's awesome.)

I'm going to take you through my routines and simple makeup and hair looks, so no matter how crazy your life is you can find some beauty in it. So put down the excuses and pick up the mascara!

BEAUTY EVOLUTION

My life in beauty began, naturally, with my mom. I started by watching Mama in the mirror, applying the same perfect cat-eye every single day.

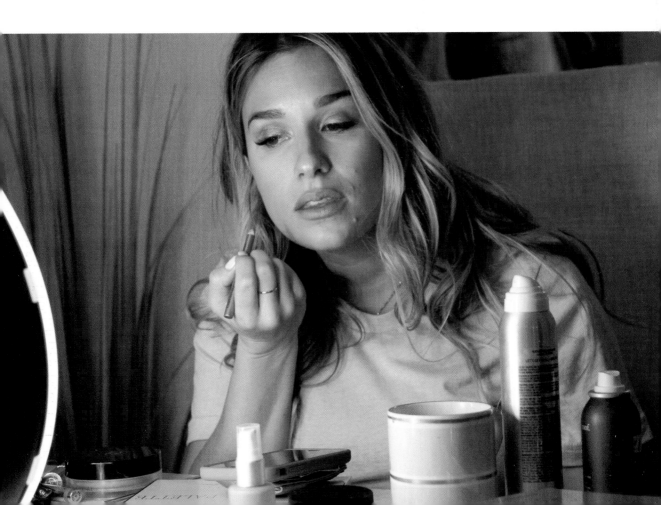

She's very good at her makeup, and we have the same eye shape, so I learned from her how starting the line closer to the inner eye or farther out can really change the look of your whole face. Everyone's face is different, and different styles and techniques can help achieve the right look for you. Luckily Mama and I look so much alike that all I had to do was watch her to get the idea of what to do early on.

As a young girl, I felt so confident at home with my mother telling us how beautiful we were all the time. But it didn't always connect at school. Growing up, other kids used to make fun of me for my thick eyebrows and moles. About my moles, they used to come up to me and say, "You have crumbs all over your face." Or they called my thick eyebrows "manly." The comments are too many to remember. There was nothing I could do about the moles, but with my eyebrows, I overtweezed them and applied yellow eye shadow to try to lighten them up. Not a great look.

At home, my mom would always tell me how beautiful my features were. "You've got eyebrows like Brooke Shields. Don't touch them."

"What about my moles?" I cried.

"Cindy Crawford has moles."

Thank God I listened to Mama, not just in terms of my self-esteem, but also my eyebrows! Thick brows are now in style, and I get complimented on mine all the time.

Out of high school and in my early twenties, I really got my beauty groove on and learned what looked best and all the techniques and tricks, thanks to my best friend and makeup artist, Jess, who always has a new tip or product for me to try. In addition to knowing how to apply products, after I met Eric, I also had the natural glow of love. But then I became a mom myself, and my beauty regimen went from a full-blown part of my life to basically nonexistent. Pre-kids, I used to get my nails done every week, my eyelashes filled regularly, spray tans, you name it. When we lived in Denver I was pampering myself weekly.

jessie says

make primping for date night part of the fun

Prepping for a night out is a good moment to transition from being a harried mom to a sexy woman. But you've got to set the mood. If Eric and I are going on a date night, I'll have a glass of wine and play some music while I'm putting on my makeup. I love this time, when I can smell Eric putting on his cologne, because it's full of anticipation. When you're getting ready, have your man pour you a glass of wine, put on your favorite music, spray your perfume, and, most of all, have fun.

Now? My nails are chipped. Facials, forget it. I spray myself with self-tanner in the shower stall. I can't remember what the inside of a spa looks like. Don't get me wrong, I could do all this stuff if I wanted, if I hired nannies to watch my children while all I did was focus on my appearance. But that's not my style.

Once in a while, I do take some real time for myself to "recharge my beauty batteries," as I call it. Sometimes you've just gotta do it, whether it's because you need a self-esteem boost or just time for yourself. That's when I tell Eric I need the afternoon, and I'll go get my nails done, lashes, spray tan, the full menu. If I haven't hit a moment of true desperation (usually the case), I'll plan it around nap time so I don't feel like I'm missing out on anything. Either way, when it gets to the point that my beauty batteries are dead, I just have to go.

EVERYDAY AND EVENT MAKEUP LOOKS

MY GO-TO DAYTIME LOOK

My daytime look varies. Sometimes I wake up and put nothing on at all. Other days I may put on tinted moisturizer and some illuminator and a coat of mascara and call it a day. If I don't want to "scare little children," as I jokingly say, then I wear a full face of makeup that appears to be "makeup-less."

PRODUCTS

Honest Beauty Younger Face Deep Hydration Cream

BECCA Shimmering Skin Perfector Pressed Highlighter (I use it in Opal)

Anastasia Beverly Hills Perfect Brow Pencil

Anastasia Beverly Hills Clear Brow Gel

Stila Convertible Color cream blush

The Jessie Decker Palette (I use my own JJD eye shadow palette, but I also like Stila's Eyes Are the Window Shadow Palette in Soul.)

FACE Atelier Ultra Foundation (I use #7 Tan)

AmazingCosmetics concealer (I use medium)

L'Oreal Paris Voluminous Original Mascara in Carbon Black

Burt's Bees lip balm

HERE'S WHAT I DO

First I moisturize my entire face.

I use my Beautyblender sponge to apply illuminator all over my face for that fresh dewy look.

After that, I use my Beautyblender again to sponge on some foundation.

Next I fill in my brows a little bit with a pencil and brush them with clear gel to hold them in place. (They are long and wild and have a mind of their own.)

I apply a nude eye shadow from my palette all over my lids. Then I dust a little shimmer gold shadow on top of my lids to make my eyes pop.

Then I apply some concealer with a brush to take away those sleepy dark circles under my eyes.

Using my finger, I dab cream blush on the apples of my cheeks while smiling.

Next I do a couple coats of mascara and apply a little lip balm.

Last, I go back over my nose and cheekbones with the illuminator sponge I used in the beginning to give my face that extra glow. I do it every time!

MY FAVE RED-CARPET LOOK

PRODUCTS

Anastasia Beverly Hills eye shadow in Birkin

NARS Isolde Duo EyeShadow

Laura Mercier Caviar Stick Eye Colour

Stila Smudge Stick Waterproof Eyeliner in Lionfish

Stila Smudge Pot black liner

Marc Jacobs Dew Drops Coconut Gel Highlighter

FACE Atelier Ultra Foundation

AmazingCosmetics concealer

Soleil Tan de Chanel bronzing makeup base

Charlotte Tilbury Beach Stick bronzer in Ibiza

Charlotte Tilbury Beach Stick bronzer in Moon Beach

Charlotte Tilbury Bar of Gold illuminating highlighter

TATCHA Luminous Dewy Skin Mist

Kopari Coconut Sheer Oil on body

Jessie Decker Lip Kit for lips

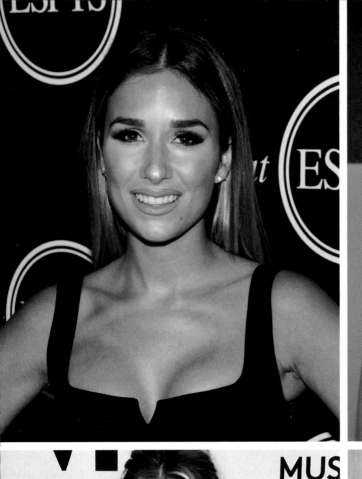
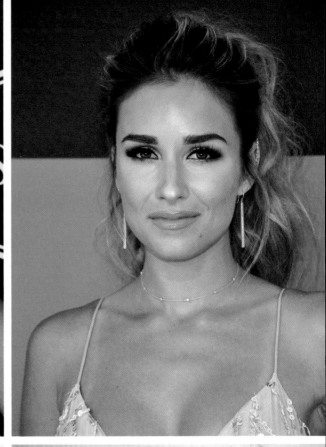
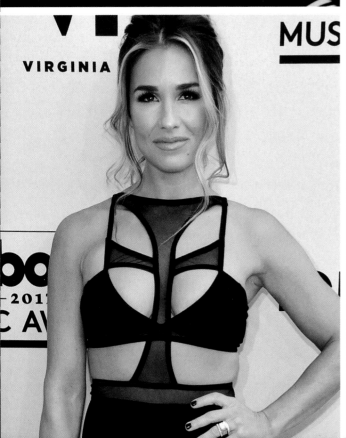
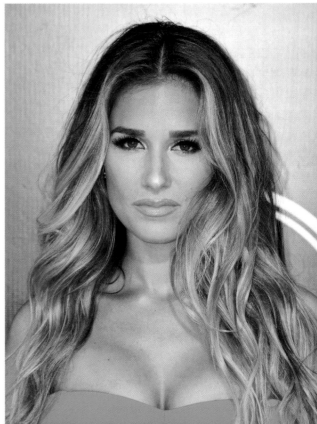

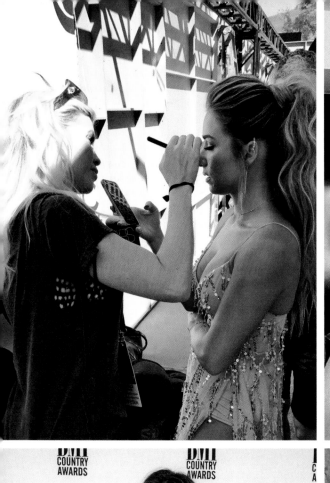

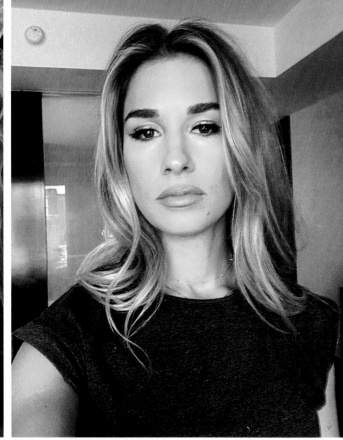

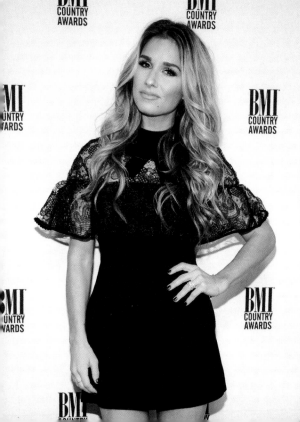

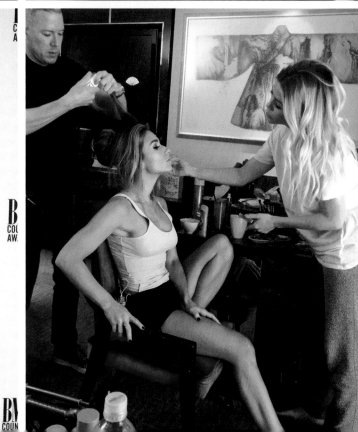

JESSICA'S DIRECTIONS

"This look is good for anyone!" says Jessica, my best friend and makeup artist who always does my look for really big events. "That's because the eye colors are great for everyone. They produce a subtle look that every eye color and skin tone can rock. The metallics pick up beautifully in photos. I do not powder Jessie, as she likes it youthful—dewy and fresh. Most girls will need to powder lightly, especially if they have oily skin. Jessie does not, so that's why we can get away with no powder. If you want powder, I recommend NARS Light Reflecting Pressed Setting Powder. For oily

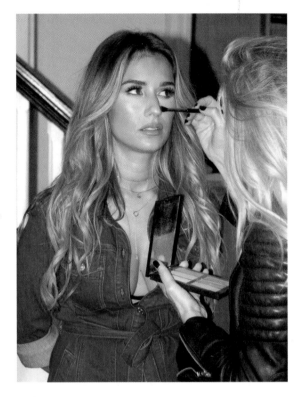

skin, try Kat Von D Lock-It Setting Powder to help makeup last longer. Also, skip the illuminating cream (Charlotte Tilbury Bar of Gold) and opt for a powder highlighter like BECCA Shimmering Skin Perfector Pressed Highlighter in Champagne Pop."

1. Prep under the eyes with Klorane Smoothing and Relaxing under-eye patches to help de-puff and keep concealer smooth.

2. Apply Smashbox 24 Hour Photo Finish Shadow Primer all over the lids.

3. Apply Anastasia Birkin eye shadow all over the lids, past the crease, and buff in small circles with brushes like Elaina Badro Blending Eye Brush.

4. With a small fluffy brush (I use Say Me 2.3 flat blending brush),

apply NARS Isolde shadow (the shimmering copper side) in the crease from the outer corners to the inner corners. Use a windshield wiper motion to create a deeper crease. Apply until you have your desired intensity of color.

5. Apply Laura Mercier Caviar Stick Eye Colour in Copper on the lids, and then set with the NARS Isolde frosted gold color over it and into the inner corners.

6. Apply the same shadow stick halfway under the lower lash lines from the inner corners to the middle of the lash lines and set with the same gold shadow used on your lids.

7. Line upper lash lines with Stila Smudge Stick Waterproof Eyeliner in Lionfish, and also line the lower lash lines from the outer corners to the halfway mark, meeting where you placed the gold.

8. Take the copper bronze color from the NARS palette and buff in the Stila eyeliner in Lionfish to meet the gold under the lower lash lines, so it's a nice fade from copper to gold and gives more of a worn-in look.

9. Apply Stila Smudge Pot black liner to create Jessie's signature eyeliner. Marc Jacobs's liquid liner is an easier option when doing your own makeup.

10. Remove the under-eye pads and clean up any fallout.

11. Prep the skin with moisturizer and Marc Jacobs Dew Drops! If you have oily skin, skip this step and proceed to foundation. This is a very dewy look, so if you feel like the illuminating cream is too much, only apply it to the cheekbones.

12. Apply FACE Atelier Ultra Foundation in shade #7 (tan) with Marc Jacobs face brush #2.

13. Apply AmazingCosmetics concealer in medium golden under the eyes and around the nose and buff in.

14. Apply Soleil Tan de Chanel bronzing makeup base around the forehead and under the cheekbones to help give a natural tan.

15. Go over the same places you just used the Chanel bronzing makeup with Charlotte Tilbury Beach Stick bronzer in Ibiza for a more defined and bronze look.

16. Add Charlotte Tilbury Beach Stick bronzer in Moon Beach on the apples of the cheeks with your fingers and tap to melt it into the skin and give a natural flush.

17. Top with Charlotte Tilbury Bar of Gold highlighter on the cheekbones and the tip of the nose. Always shine that nose, girls!

18. Apply Ardell individual lashes for a natural soft look.

19. Finish by spraying TATCHA Luminous Dewy Skin Mist.

DRUGSTORE CHEAT SHEET

If you're on a budget, swap out some of the pricier products above for these drugstore finds!

Pix! Eye Reflection Shadow Palette replaces the Nars shadow

COVERGIRL Queen Collection major shade liquid lipstick in Insider replaces Jessie's lip kit

Katy Perry COVERGIRL Katy Kat gloss in Cateloupe over the lipstick that replaces Jessie's lip kit

COVERGIRL liquid liner in shade 325 (black) replaces Stila Smudge Pot or Marc Jacobs liner

COVERGIRL Vitalist Healthy Concealer replaces AmazingCosmetics

COVERGIRL Vitalist Healthy Glow Highlighter in shade 6 can be used on eyes instead of the Laura Mercier shadow stick

COVERGIRL TruBLEND matte for girls who have oily skin

L'Oréal Paris True Match Lumi Glotion replaces Marc Jacobs Dew Drops if you have drier skin

Skintreats Pixi Glow Mist replaces Tatcha Luminous Dewy Skin Mist

JESSIE'S NIGHTTIME BEAUTY ROUTINE

* I bathe every night after the kids go down to sleep. I don't *ever* skip it. I'm super weird about that. Sometimes I shower, but usually I take a bath. (I love LIERAC Paris Hydra Body Scrub to exfoliate.) I'm a bath person. It's something special to look forward to. I light candles and listen to music or read a book. Sometimes Eric comes in the bath with me, but if not, I have a chair next to my bathtub, and we just talk. That's our time.

* I wash my face with good old soap and water. Literally a bar of soap or a body scrub to exfoliate my face. I'm not sure that's the best advice, but that's what I do. It comes from the fact that my skin is so sensitive that it doesn't tolerate a lot of fancy cleansers.

* After cleansing, I always moisturize. Once a week I put on a clear hydrating mask that you sleep in, because I have very dry skin. I love Boscia Tsubaki Deep Hydration Sleeping Mask. It's the best and smells amazing.

* When I go to bed, I look like a grease ball. That's because from

jessie says
what every girl needs

Everyone needs a robe—or three. I have all kinds of robes. Soft cotton. Really thick, fuzzy ones for the winter. Towel robes for when you get out of the shower. I live in robes and really comfy slippers while I'm doing my makeup.

I've been blessed with good skin, so I'm not going to sell you on what to do to have good skin. That wouldn't be fair. Genetics have a ton to do with it. What I will say is because I have very dry skin, I never get pimples or acne. But I have to constantly exfoliate the dry dead skin and then apply oils or other moisturizers. If I get a pimple or a blemish, then I know it's my skin lacking vitamin D. I will head straight to the tanning salon. UV rays have been proven to cause skin damage, but I'm not suggesting a weekly appointment. This is just a case-by-case situation. When I lie on the tanning bed, those blemishes or pimples go away. Because Eric gets acne sometimes from all the sweat and oil that playing football produces, I have him do it too, and it clears up his skin as well.

the neck down, I slather on Eucerin lotion. It's worth it, though. Anyone who ever touches my skin compliments me on its softness. I think it's because I hydrate the heck out of it.

JESSIE'S MORNING BEAUTY ROUTINE

In the morning, I wash off my mask and put on a tinted moisturizer. On the days I don't feel like doing a lot of makeup, I put on a little under-eye concealer, sponge on some cream blush, brush and gel my eyebrows (they can look crazy in the morning because they're so long), apply a little Burt's Bees lip balm, throw on a "vavoom" ponytail, and that's it.

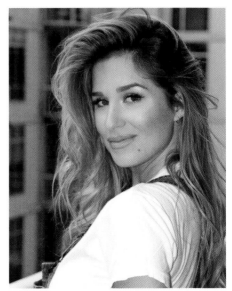

JESSIE'S HAIR ROUTINE

I have to start out with a subject I'm passionate about: big hair! I've always had big hair and it works for my face shape and personal style. I usually do boho waves with an iron or use hot rollers. I know rollers are something that have gone out of style, but they should never be out of style. I'll put my head in a full set of hot rollers and do my makeup. Once I take it out, dip my head over, and spray the whole thing, trust me, it looks amazing. It's so easy. Instead of standing there and curling each piece one by one, you put your whole head in hot rollers and are done with it.

When I do my hair, it lasts for a few days. So many mornings I don't touch it. But because my hair gets greasy fast, I spray tons of dry shampoo in it. I think every girl should keep dry shampoo and a teaser comb on her, just to keep her hair looking full. There's nothing worse than having really stringy, flat hair.

I'll do a hydrating mask on my hair once a month. If I don't have anything to do the next day, I'll smother my hair in coconut oil, sleep on it, and then pile my hair into a baseball hat so it can marinate the entire day. There's nothing like it for shiny, healthy hair.

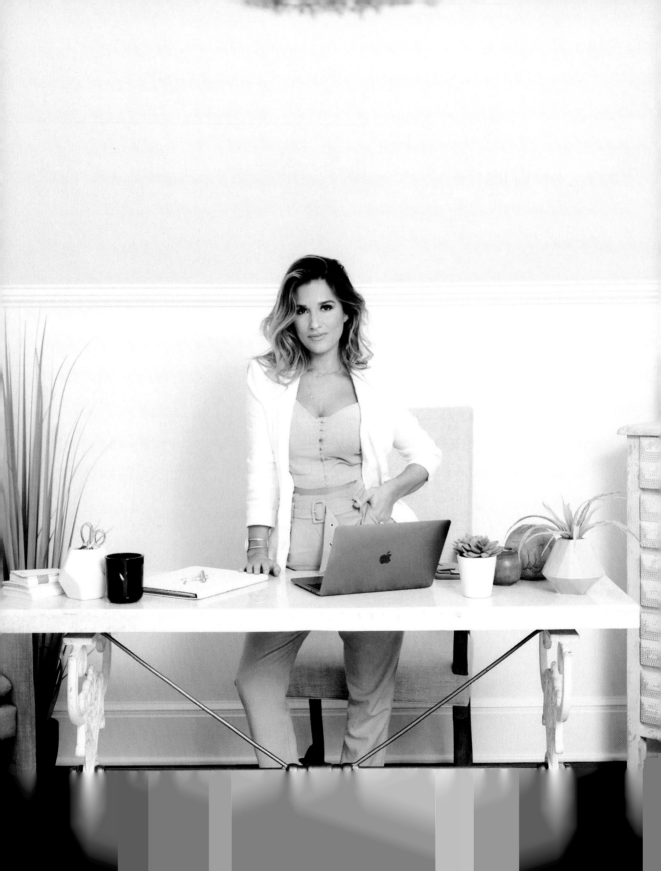

fashion for me

I've always loved fashion, even as a kid. When I was in high school, I wasn't afraid to experiment with my look. I'm talking fuzzy boots and leopard-print pants. I was all over the place.

While the other kids around me only wanted to be preppy, dressing in head-to-toe Abercrombie & Fitch, I wanted to dress like a celebrity. Fascinated by Hollywood style, I closely followed what singers like Britney Spears, Jessica Simpson, and Shakira wore. I'd even make my own clothes when I couldn't find the latest trends I wanted to try out. I was adventurous and into being unique—while still looking cute, of course.

Even though I'm now grown up and have kids of my own, essentially my approach to clothes isn't all that different. My look is still eclectic and trendy, and still true to me. Like most women, I find inspiration for new ideas by checking out fashion magazines, websites, and Instagram feeds. I always think it's best when experimenting, however, to remember what's flattering for my body. Just because something is in style does not mean it looks good on everybody. When I'm not pregnant, I have a typical gymnast's body—petite, muscular, and not a ton of curves. I always put flattering before anything else.

No matter whether I'm being a southern belle or a boho babe, my philosophy is the same: style is just another way of expressing your creativity.

jessie says
let kids be kids—even when it comes to their clothes

I get most of my kids' clothes from Target or Amazon. You don't need to spend a lot of money on fancy children's clothes. There's no point. They mess them up—as they should. Kids are kids. I think it's weird when I see children all dressed up in stiff or mature outfits. They just want to be comfortable. Don't we all? But with children, who are constantly moving around, ease is more important than anything else. Half the time my kids are in their pajamas, even when we go out places. I don't care. When Vivi (whose hair is always wild and messy) wanted to wear her pajamas and rain boots last night out to dinner, I said, "She looks cute. Let her be."

KITTENISH

I described myself as an adventurous dresser when I was a kid, but I'm bolder now than I have ever been when it comes to my style. That's because I'm more confident now than I've ever been in every aspect of my life. I've come into my own, not only as a woman, but also as a designer!

Since I was fifteen years old, I wanted to have my own clothing line—and I knew if I did, it would be called Kittenish. The name came to me when I was still a teen, after a woman told me I was very "kittenish." Loving the sound and idea, I filed it away for the future. Meanwhile, I was always sketching outfits. Even while in math class when I should have been focusing on numbers, I was drawing clothes.

Fast-forward through the beginning of my music career and getting married: I finally had the courage to find a partner and launch Kittenish. It debuted in the summer of 2015 with only five pieces. Each was a true reflection of my own taste and style. There was, of course, a flannel shirt and cutoff short shorts. But there was also a cute floral romper (as well as a black lacy one) and a stunning black bandage dress. I designed a line of exactly the kind of clothes I would wear—and they all sold out.

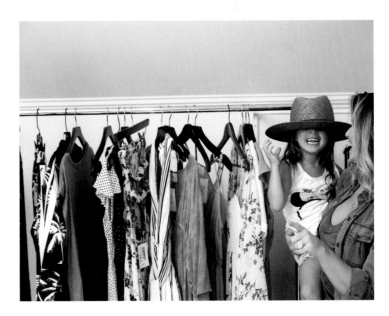

The thing I love about fashion is it's just so cut-and-dried. People either like it or they don't. They either want to buy the clothes or they don't want to. There isn't politics like *jessie says*

fashion must-haves

There are definitely key items that you need to have in your closet, whatever body type or lifestyle you have. I suggest investing a little more in these staples, even if most of them aren't flashy or statement pieces, since you'll return to them over and over again. I couldn't live without a single one.

* **A PAIR OF NUDE PUMPS.** They elongate your legs. Being short, I wear mine all the time.

* **A BASEBALL CAP.** Throw one on and everyone'll think you're cool—not having a bad hair day.

* **HIGH-QUALITY LEGGINGS.** I have a whole bunch of them, because I live in them.

* **A CRISP WHITE V-NECK.** This is just sexy, easy, and goes with absolutely everything. It's an especially good piece when you're traveling and want to pack light.

* **AVIATOR SUNGLASSES.** These are classic and look great on every face shape.

* **CUTOFF JEANS.** I came out of my mama wearing these. JK! But I probably have three hundred pairs of these. They're a southern-girl staple.

* **SNEAKERS.** I love me some sneakers—they make anything immediately cute and flirty.

* **A SLOUCHY, OFF-THE-SHOULDER SWEATER.** There's nothing more irresistible than the look of a soft sweater that shows a bit of shoulder.

* **A FUN PAIR OF HEELS THAT ARE JUST WILD.** I have a pair with fuzz all over the strap that I'll throw on with a pair of rolled-up blue jeans and a T-shirt for a casual outfit with a pop of Carrie Bradshaw.

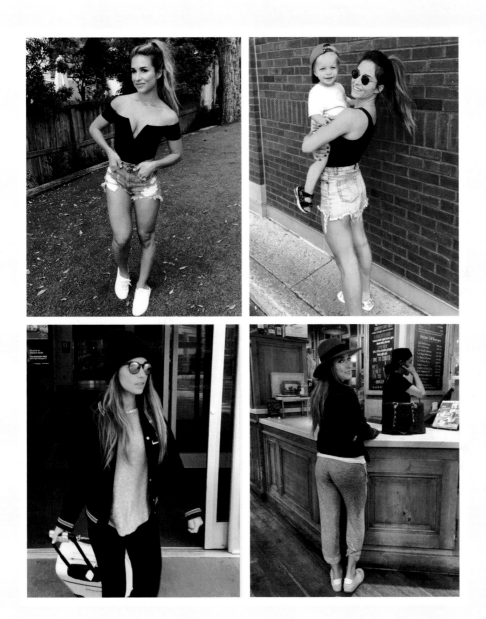

* **A LEATHER JACKET.** This can edge up any look.

* **A BEANIE FOR THE WINTER.** This can turn you into an instant star. Everyone will take notice if you pair your beanie with a leather jacket and aviators. You will have people thinking a rock star just walked into the room.

there is in show business. After its debut line, Kittenish doubled in sales, then tripled, until it grew into the multimillion-dollar clothing company it is today. And that's due to the fact that I know my customers. It's so easy, because they are just like me. This was proved to me when I went through a phase where I wasn't as hands-on with the styles. I had just had Bubby and, overwhelmed, I needed a break. Well, those items didn't sell. That was the moment when I really found out I needed my hand in every detail, because I really understand my fans and customers.

RED-CARPET READY

Picking out a red-carpet look is always a fiasco for me. Every. Single. Time. I always wait till there are just days to spare and I'm overnighting something from Revolve or Jessica is calling in last-minute favors from stylists or designers. I have no sense of time or urgency. It always kind of works out, and I rely on that. Most celebs or people in the public eye have a stylist who pulls hundreds of looks, shoes, and jewelry and sets them up in a room where they get styled. Oh, and that costs them around $7,000 to $10,000 a night when all is said and done! I just can't fathom spending that for one night. I know that doesn't sound very "celeb," but maybe that's the frugal girl from Georgia in me. I have literally walked the carpet in a look that cost fifty bucks and rocked it! I style it with some fancy shoes and great hair and makeup, and it always turns out great.

RED-CARPET HITS AND MISSES

THE 51ST ACADEMY OF COUNTRY MUSIC AWARDS IN LAS VEGAS (2016)

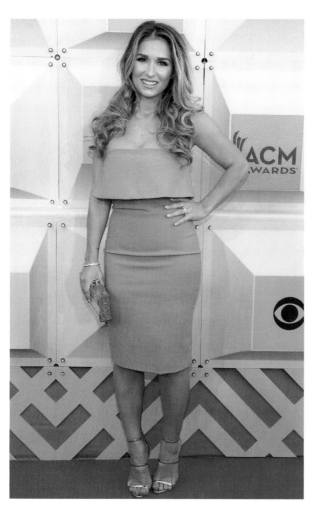

This is my least-favorite red-carpet look. I'm always last minute, but I got this pink dress in the last second. We were also super rushed getting my hair and makeup ready. I only had Jessica for makeup and no one for my hair. I just couldn't get my hair right! (Probably because nothing else was working.) I wasn't in the shape I wanted to be in and just felt uncomfortable the entire time. With my toes poking out of my shoes, my feet were killing me so badly that in the middle of the awards show I texted Jessica to go find me more comfortable shoes. God bless her—she did, at Aldo, and I swapped them out in the middle of the awards ceremony!

THE 2016 ESPYS

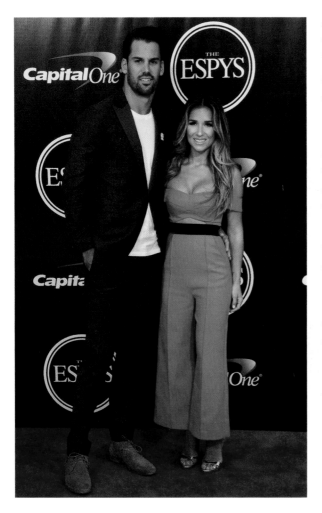

My favorite red-carpet moment was a red jumpsuit I wore to the ESPYS. I had originally picked out another dress, but the morning of the sports awards ceremony I decided to go to Robertson Boulevard in LA, and as I walked down the street I looked in the window of Intermix and saw the cutest outfit on the mannequin. "I'm grabbing that!" I said to myself. I went in and tried it on, grabbed a pair of shoes to match, and that was the outfit! I picked my red-carpet look an hour before I was supposed to get ready! Jessica did my makeup (of course), and Rick Henry, who is my go-to hair guy, did a fabulous job. That's probably the prettiest I've ever felt on the red carpet.

THE 52ND ACADEMY OF COUNTRY MUSIC
AWARDS IN LAS VEGAS (2017)

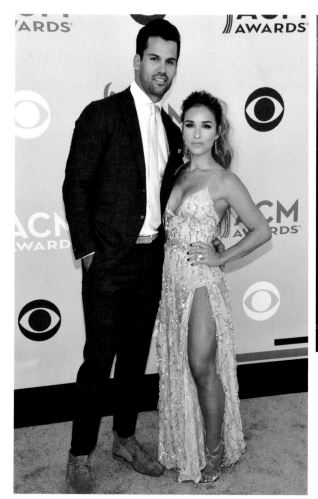

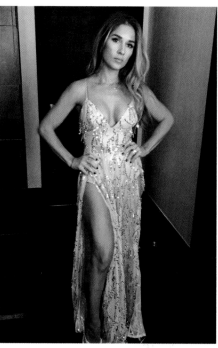

Not only was I walking it, but I was also cohosting the red carpet for Dick Clark Productions, so you would assume I would've been better prepared. Ha! I wore a beautiful gold dress that was supposed to be Jessica's reception dress at her wedding (she decided against it, but held on to it). I had nothing to wear, naturally, and she had brought it in her carry-on bag. As soon as she arrived at the hotel, we ran into the lobby bathroom and I tried on the dress and knew immediately it was the one. We paired it with gorgeous Chloe makeup. Rick had the idea of doing a sassy ponytail. That's another fave.

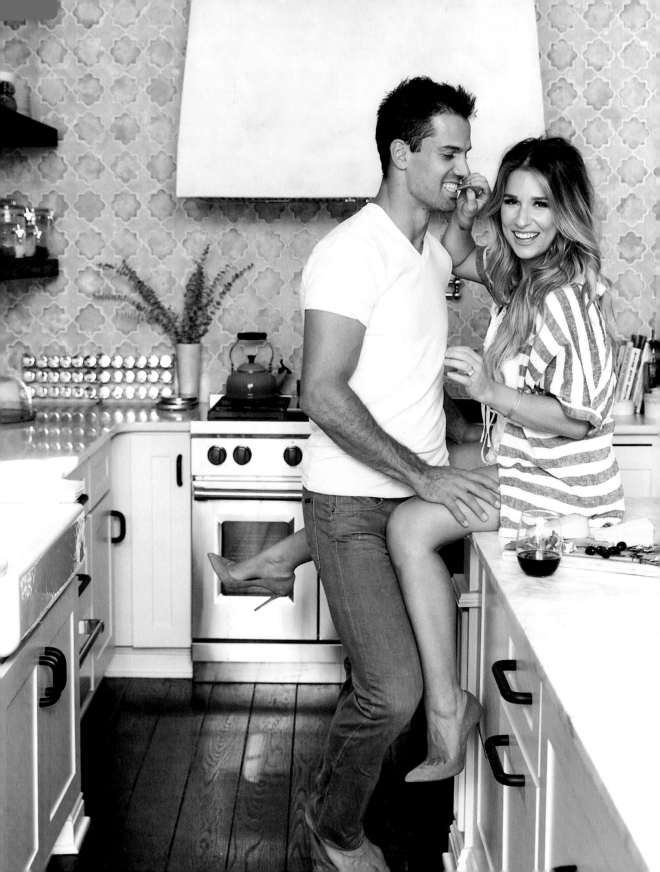

making the fairy tale work

Eric and I have a pact during football season that I try to tone down my work as much as possible to be his support system. I'm like a '50s housewife, having dinner warm and ready when he returns home, massaging his back, taking care of him in any and every way. But as soon as football's over, it's my turn. I get to go on tour, travel, and be creative, while Eric is the first-responder parent. I'm lucky to have a man who is happy to take on a fifty-fifty parent partnership, and I try to take full advantage of that time.

Motherhood has made me more driven and conscious of my time. I get more done because work is always put into the perspective of my family. Recently, I canceled a morning meeting in the city because Bubby threw up in the car and Vivi was a little clingy. "Is this meeting important enough that I need to be away from the babies?" I asked myself. And it wasn't. It hardly ever is.

It's impossible not to feel guilty as a mom (unless, as I said, you're not a good mom: those are the only ones who think they do everything perfectly). I have those moments too, and not because I'm a working mom, but because I am always trying to live up to the example of my own mom. While I was growing up, she worked—and I mean supported-a-family kind of worked. She woke us up every morning smiling and cheery and made us breakfast; she was ready with snacks when we got home from school; and she regularly prepared us five-course dinners and then put all of us to bed. That is no exaggeration.

I'm always trying to live up to those high expectations of what it means to be a working mom. There's one moment from my childhood that pretty much sums it all up. I was too sick to go to school, but my mom, who was hosting a TV show, had to go to work. She was the on-air talent. She didn't have anyone to watch me, so she had to take me to work. As I got out of the car in the parking lot, I threw up, and my mom patted my back sweetly. There was nothing else she could do. We had no family around; my dad was gone and she was totally on her own. Yet, bundled up with a Sprite and crackers, watching my pretty mom doing her hosting job on set, I felt totally cared for.

Sometimes women get this idea in their heads that they have to choose whether to be a mommy or a career woman. I love being a mother, but I also think it's important to have something for yourself. I feel very proud of what I contribute to my family as a provider. I don't have to; financially, I could stay at home, but that would make me crazy. Some women don't feel that way, but my career is part of how I find my worth.

For those of you who feel like I do, I'm living proof that you can do both. I just drink a lot of coffee. Oh, and I married a great partner. I could never do any of this without Eric.

My hubby and I have never had any major fights: no yelling or name-calling. We don't fight that way. He definitely can get a little grumpy when I'm gone working a lot. He's just happier when I'm home and around. I get it. I'm the same way; I want him around.

Although he says he doesn't like me working so much, he's a big reason for my success—and not just because he's a great dad. Eric gives me confidence and even pushes me in my career. When I was twenty weeks pregnant with Forrest, I was asked to cohost the American Music Awards red-carpet coverage in Los Angeles for Dick Clark Productions and take part in the radio remotes. It was a big deal, but I had just returned from a business trip to New York City the week before, and by that point in my pregnancy, I had said I wasn't going to travel anymore. Plus Eric had three days off, which we were planning on spending together.

I was all set to turn it down, but Eric talked me into going. "Selfishly, I

ERIC SAYS

BRING HOME THE BACON!

I wish she were at home all the time, because I like to be taken care of. But in the bigger picture, I love that she pursues her dreams and challenges herself. We always joke that once I retire, she's going to be the sugar mama and I'm going to be a stay-at-home dad. It's perfect, because I'm a homebody, and I love having a family.

want you to stay. But this is a great opportunity," he said. "I've got the kids. You go ahead."

He is such a good man.

WORKING MOMS

Remember the episode of *Sex and the City* when Miranda had to quit her big job at the law firm? Well, if you don't, she left because she got sick of explaining to her boss where she was going when she was doing stuff for her kid. Unfortunately, a lot of offices aren't that friendly to moms. That's one of the reasons being an entrepreneur is such an important option for women. I have a girlfriend who runs her own interior decorating business and has a whole bunch of kids. She came over to my house with her baby on her hip and pointed to where I should install the curtains. She's a total badass.

I love working from home, because even if you're not able to be on top of your children all day, you are still around—and the kids love that. Today, I worked from home and Bubby was here. I was on the phone doing an interview and then had a big planning session with my team about my upcoming schedule, but he was happy because he knew Mommy was in the same house.

Being your own boss can be really great, but it's far from easy. The tradeoff is that you have to make all the decisions and are responsible for everything. I've learned a few lessons along the way that I want all my ladies to know:

* **RECOGNIZE GOOD PEOPLE CAN COME FROM ANYWHERE.** I met my manager, Matt Musacchio, at a show I was playing in Syracuse with my first label. He was in the meet-and-greet line to get his

album signed and take a picture with me. He was a huge fan of mine! Little did I know that ten years later he'd be my manager. (He contacted me through MySpace, came on as an intern, and worked his way up.) I've gone through five managers, and Matt is the best. Not only is he brilliant (he was valedictorian of his high school class and has a law degree), but he really loves music. I'm certain we will be friends forever.

* **NOT EVERYONE IS GOING TO LIKE YOU.** I've struggled a lot in the music industry and still to this day I have to keep proving myself. But that doesn't mean I'm ever going to stop doing things my way.

* **TRY NOT TO GET VISIBLY EMOTIONAL ABOUT WORK MATTERS.** I say this not because there's anything wrong with emotion, but because if you do, people will focus more on you being emotional than the issue at hand. Be clear. Be articulate. If you're upset or unhappy with something, try instead to say, "This isn't working for me, and we need to find a solution." People will respond better that way.

MY SECRETS TO A SUCCESSFUL MARRIAGE

BE A TEAM AT ALL TIMES

No one should ever *win* an argument in a marriage. If someone wins, that means someone else loses. Eric and I are a team a hundred percent of the time, so if he wins, I win, and vice versa. I don't want Eric to ever feel like he is not heard.

It helps that we have similar views on three subjects that I think are crucial for couples to agree on for a successful, long-lasting marriage.

They are, not surprisingly, money, politics, and religion. If you don't agree on these major building blocks to a life (something you should figure out while still dating), there will be trouble down the road. I've witnessed that in my own life and with many of my friends. When you bring children into the world, any conflicts will only become more complicated.

Eric and I share identical viewpoints on the Big Three. It's part of what attracted us to each other. Not that we always express ourselves similarly. Take money, for example. I'm a spender, and he is a saver. But our basic approach to finances is on the same wavelength. Although we both came from humble beginnings, neither of us feels compelled to show off our wealth by being covered in labels or throwing over-the-top parties. We like to drive nice cars and live stylishly and comfortably, but that's about it. So our different natures regarding money complement each other—Eric helps me be responsible while I help him enjoy himself.

COMMUNICATION IS KEY

The majority of men I know have a hard time expressing themselves and don't feel comfortable pouring their hearts out, which makes good emotional communication a challenge. However, there are certain things you can do to set yourself up for success when talking with your guy.

Nobody responds well to extreme drama. Crying intensely or screaming is not a good way to get your point across. Speak in a calm manner. I will do things like put my hand on top of Eric's hand and lightly rub it. Then I will calmly look him in the eye and say, "I would really like for you to hear what I'm saying." That's much more effective than a shouting match.

When I can finally get Eric to open up, I like to reinforce that he is doing a great job so that he'll talk more. I do that by telling him outright that I hear him, understand how he feels, and respect his opinion. Or I pull the old counselor trick and ask, "How did that make you feel?" It's a nice open-ended question a guy can answer however they want to.

There's nothing Eric hates more than when I repeatedly ask him, "What's wrong?" A lot of times, I don't think he knows what's bothering him. Sometimes I will study him and then run through a few things that might be issues, but mostly I give him the space to express himself when he's ready.

MAINTAIN A BALANCE

Eric and I don't need to be up in each other's grill 24/7. We need our space and want that for each other. We are so confident in our relationship that it gives us freedom.

Eric and I take time for ourselves even if we are in the same house. I might be sitting in my room working on my computer as the baby nurses, while he's downstairs in the movie theater, decompressing by watching a show. It's nice to be together and apart at the same time.

However, we also snatch little moments to connect. You don't need to wait for date night (with three kids, those are hard to come by these days). Even if it's only ten minutes, that's enough to look at each other and say, "Hey, I like you." For Eric and me, our connection time is often over afternoon lattes. I make a beautiful coffee that I serve him, and then we sit on the back porch together, sipping delicious drinks and chatting while we watch our kids playing. What could be better? (Well, the other night we popped open a bottle of prosecco and enjoyed it in the tub while the baby was in his carrier. That was pretty fun.)

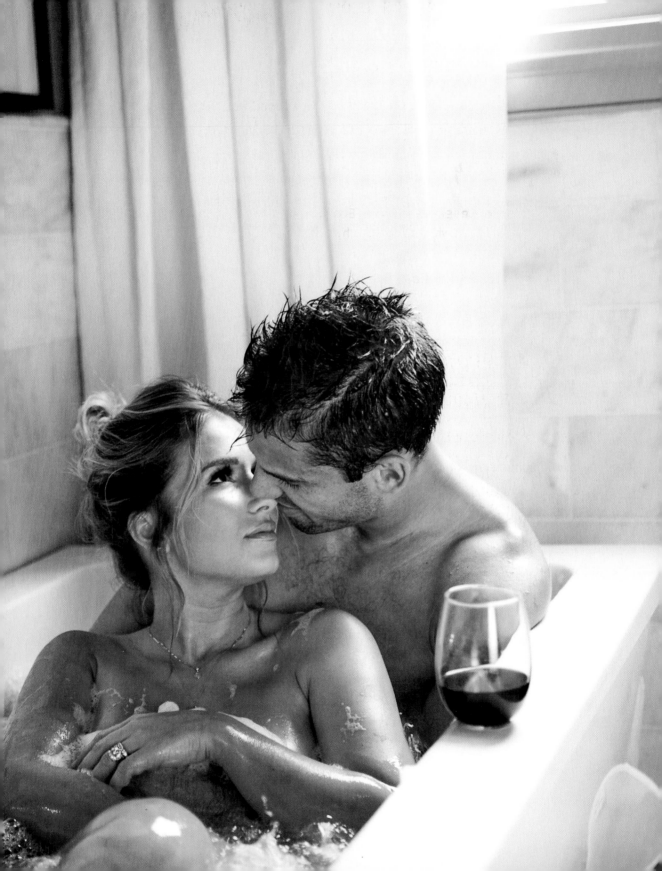

keep it sexy

* **KEEP YOURSELF GROOMED.** Even though you get comfortable with your partner, when it comes to hygiene, act like you've been dating your husband for a month, max.

* **LOOK, NOBODY GOES TO SLEEP IN A FULL SET OF LINGERIE.** Come on. Let's get real. But I still like Eric to see what I've got going on. So, although sometimes I'll wear the full PJ set, usually I go to sleep in a T-shirt and underwear. Casual but revealing. Perfect.

* **BE PLAYFUL AND SILLY.** Eric and I have a running joke where one of us will get into bed totally naked and pull the covers up to the neck so that when the other one gets in, it's like, "Oh, hello!" The surprise is a little bit sexy but also kind of funny. The other day while I was trying to get work done in a rare moment of the baby napping, Eric, who was walking from the laundry room to the living room, pulled his pants down and showed it off. He was just being silly to bring a little lightness to our lives as working parents of young children.

* **TOUCH IS THERAPEUTIC.** Eric and I always give each other massages—every night—even if it's only for five minutes. Physical touch is so important. But we aren't big snugglers in bed. That makes us feel suffocated. While we sleep, we just touch feet!

STAYING FRONT AND CENTER
WITH YOUR FAMILY

It's really important for your kids to connect *you* with the things you do for them, whether it's making the lunch in their lunch box, putting up decorations for the holidays, or giving them their nightly bath.

"This is for you," I say when I hand anything I've cooked for my children over to them, so that even though they may not realize it, what I've made for them stays in their brain.

And this doesn't just apply to children but to your spouse as well. Early in my relationship with Eric, I made some cookies and put them on a plate for him, then handed the plate to my mother. "Here, Mom," I said casually. "Can you go give this to Eric?"

"You bring it to him," she said, "and serve it with a big old smile. He needs to see his wife doing this."

She was right, and forever after I try to make anything I bring him—coffee, a piece of cake, or a five-course-meal—a mini-event, even if that just means putting his whiskey in a chilled glass.

Moms always seem to be behind the scenes, making everything work like the Wizard of Oz. But that can be frustrating for you, as well as give your family the wrong impression that things just happen by magic. You are working hard to make sure they are well cared for, and they should understand that. Not in a martyr way—it can be done with joy. But it shouldn't be forgotten or taken for granted.

I find the best way to do this is to stay front and center in my children's lives. For example, I believe that parents should ideally be the ones to tuck their kids in every single night and wake them every single morning. The last face they see before bed and first when they wake up in the morning should be Mommy's or Daddy's.

I said "ideally," but most of us don't live in an ideal world. I have a lot of flexibility because I usually work from home. Still, there are times when I travel or have a late-night function and I *can't* be there to bathe or tuck my babies in, so my mom or sister will take over.

This might sound crazy, but if I have been traveling, I will gently wake up my children when I get home. I don't shake them or flip on the lights and startle them. Instead, I'll rub Vivi's or Bubby's back and whisper in their little ear, "I just want you to know that Mommy's home." They go right back to sleep and sleep even better than they would have if I hadn't done that.

So to all the businesswomen working their butts off and the nurses who have to pull overnight shifts, you can make that connection with your children. It's still important (maybe even more important). Go into their rooms and create a bond through physical touch by rubbing their backs. Then whisper reassuring words: "Mommy loves you and will be home from work soon." You don't need to wake them; they can hear you anyway.

It doesn't matter what form or shape the messages you send to the ones around you take. Whether it's something as little as a note on a napkin or as grand as a huge bash marking a birthday or major milestone, the feeling is still the same—and that's love.

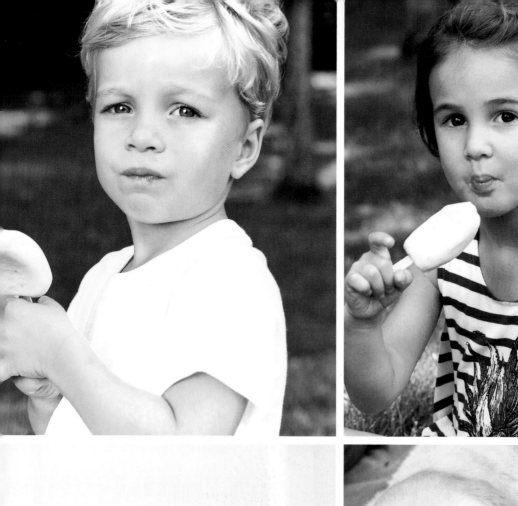
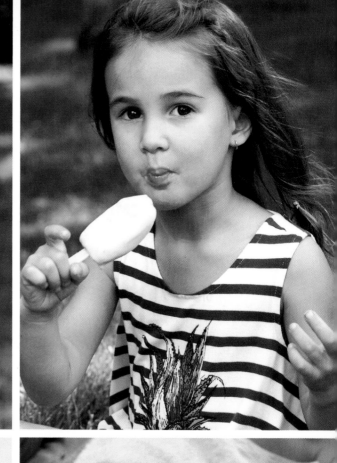
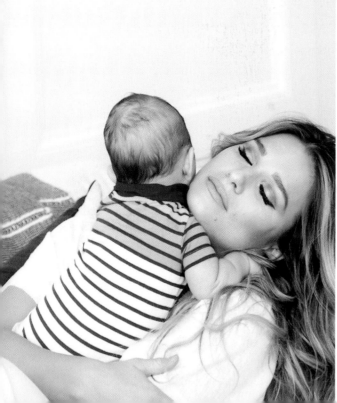
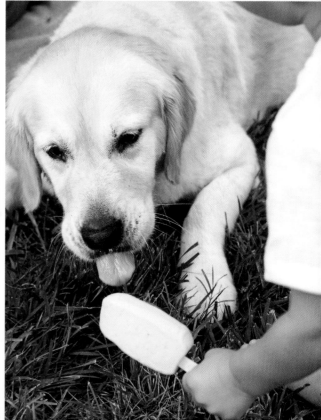

closing thoughts

What I hope y'all can take from this book is that you can do anything you put your mind to, and to dream and never stop dreaming. We all deserve the fairy tale, and we all deserve a happy life. Whether you're a college student, a single mom, a hardworking businesswoman, a loving wife, or maybe all of the above. Remember to not be hard on yourself, but to also kick some butt and go for it! My mama always says you have to see it to believe it to achieve it, and she is right. I hope my story has inspired you, given you some insight, or just hopefully made you laugh. We all have roots and a place where we began, but it's about how we choose to take the journey and what size wings we want to strap on to fly.

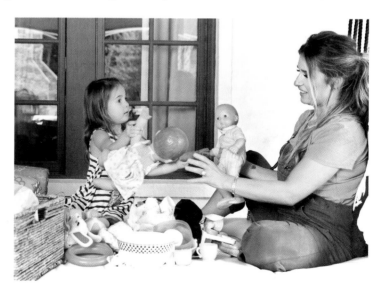

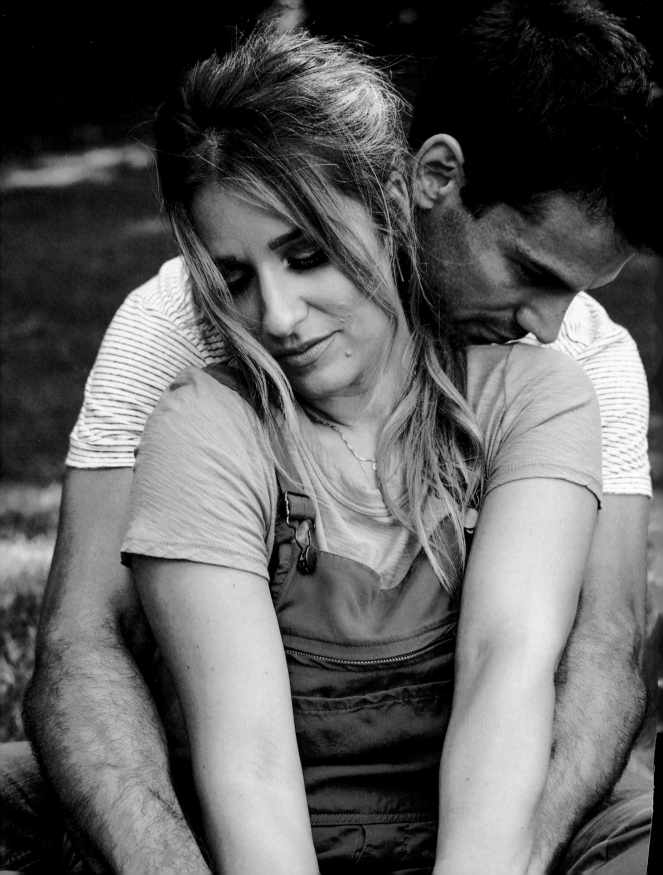

acknowledgments

This book was something I wanted to write for a long time in hopes of spreading some love, laughter, and encouragement, but I couldn't have written it without the huge support system and amazing team around me. I am beyond grateful for everyone who made this book happen.

Eric and my babies, Vivi, Bubby, and Forrest, y'all are my purpose in life, my reason, my world. Eric, you helped me become the woman I am today; your unconditional love and encouragement pushes me to be the best version of myself. I couldn't walk this world without you, my sweet soul mate. My babies, you are the greatest thing I've ever done, and my life has the most meaning and purpose because of y'all: Vivianne, my favorite girl in the whole world, always keeping me on my toes; Bubby, mommy's affectionate sweet baby boy; and little Forrest, my smiley laughing boy with the best laugh. I love being your mommy.

To my mama: without you, I wouldn't be me nor would I be where I am today. You have been my biggest supporter, my life guide, and my friend: "In a way, I owe all my creativity to her"—*Divine Secrets of the Ya-Ya Sisterhood* quote, ha! A huge thank-you for your countless hours of looking through old photos of me as a kid, being on calls with my team, and grabbing your Canon and capturing all of the beautiful photos and moments, which really helped me piece my story together. I couldn't have done it without you. Sydney, for always having my back and always being my best friend and the most loyal girl I know. John, for your constant support and encouragement and always making me laugh harder than anyone else. Steve, for being the glue in our family and the voice of reason, and for your kind heart and being an amazing dad and Paw-Paw to the babies.

I want to thank my amazing team at HarperCollins who helped step by step with this book, especially Lisa Sharkey for making this project happen and Matt Harper for his expert editing. I also want to thank my amazing agent, Lauren Nogy; my book agent, Sean Berard at APA; and my manager, Matt Musacchio, for all your help putting this project together. Rebecca Paley, thank you so much for your guidance through this process, and a huge thank-you for all the phone calls and text messages and emails to make sure my story and voice was heard. I could not have done this without you. Thank you to Meghan Prophet, my badass publicist.

Jessica Payne, my sister from another mister and best friend and amazing makeup artist (you always make me feel so pretty). Tec Petaja, thank you for all of your beautiful photography and for helping me make my story come to life through the images. A special thanks to my food stylist, Liz Schoch, for making my recipes look beautiful. Thanks to Amanda O'Connor for styling and to Katie Archer for hair on this book shoot.

Fans: y'all are what I always dreamed and hoped for as a little girl. I am so lucky to have such amazing fans like you who always have my back. You are the reason I keep going. I will always be so grateful for your endless support. Y'all "get" me and I "get" y'all right back.

photo credits

Tec Petaja: pages viii, ix, 61, 104, 110, 117, 120, 128, 129, 130, 131, 135, 138, 140, 144 (top right and bottom), 145, 149, 152, 154, 158, 164, 165, 173, 202, 205, 207, 212, 220, 224, 225, and 226.

Karen Parker: pages 3, 5, 6, 7, 8, 9, 10 (top), 15, 19, 20, 24, 26, 27 (top two images and bottom right), 29, 30, 44, 52, 55, 56, 62 (bottom), 94, 99, 107, 108, 115, 144 (bottom left), 150, 186, 189, 196, and 200.

Steve Parker: pages 16, 22 (top), and 27 (bottom left).

Avery Sports: page 28 (bottom two images).

Matt Musacchio: pages 33, 79 (middle left), and 195 (top left).

Courtesy of the author: pages 35, 93, 101 (top), 118, 137, 167, 168, 170, 172, and 195 (top right).

Jody Zorn: pages 66, 80, 88, and 89.

Eric Decker: pages 67 (top) and 103.

E! Entertainment: page 71.

Jason Ninja Williams: page 72.

Sydney Bass: pages 74 and 195 (bottom right).

Courtesy of Grand Ole Opry: pages 78 and 79 (bottom right).

Dino Gomez: page 91 (top).

Shannon Johnson: page 91 (bottom three images).

Liz Schoch: pages 133, 157, 160, 162, 166, 174, 176, 179, 181, 182, 184, and 185.

Michael Kovac: page 194 (top left).

John Shearer: pages 194 (top right and bottom left) and 211 (left).

Alberto E. Rodriguez: page 194 (bottom right).

Erika Goldring: page 195 (bottom left).

Taylor Hill: page 209.

Greg DeGuire: page 210.

Jessica Payne: page 211 (right).